COOL THE FIRE:

Curb Inflammation and Balance Hormones

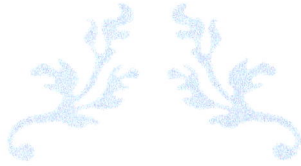

COOL THE FIRE:
CURB INFLAMMATION AND BALANCE HORMONES

28 Days to Renewed Vitality

RUTH CLARK, RD, MPH

Cooling the Fire: Curb Inflammation and Balance Hormones

by Ruth Clark, RD, MPH

Copyright ©2019 Smart Nutrition LLC

ISBN: 978-0-578-60718-4

Medical Disclaimer: This book contains advice and information relating to health care. It should be used to supplement rather than replace the advice of your doctor or another trained health professional. If you know or suspect you have a health problem, it is recommended that you seek your physician's or health care provider's advice before embarking on any medical program or treatment. All efforts have been made to assure the accuracy of the information contained in this book as of the date of publication. This publisher and the author disclaim liability for any medical outcomes that may occur as a result of applying the methods and information suggested in this book.

Table of Contents

INTRODUCTION

Are you tired of struggling with aches and pains, belly fat, brain fog, and debilitating fatigue? Do you pine for the days when you were full of vitality, inspiration and ready to take on the world?

I know exactly how it feels to be exhausted, sick too often, stressed, losing confidence and struggling with belly fat. Our bodies do start to change in mid-life, but you don't need to put up with it. I am going to be 68 years old this year and I don't feel a day older than 55. And the truth is that I felt a lot worse when I was 55. More about this later but YOU can do this, too!

In my practice, I have found that many people want to eat healthier, but they don't know how. They are stuck in a groove of eating out far too often, relying on prepackaged or unhealthy prepared fast foods and/or struggling with a sugar addiction. When they do undertake a new healthy eating plan, they are motivated for the first few days or even weeks but then succumb to cravings and hunger.

Hormones and inflammation are two big reasons why you may be struggling with your weight, exhausted all the time, or just not feeling like your old self, perhaps even suffering from anxiety or depression. But the good news is that you have profound control over your health and the aging process.

Here is why. Each of us is dealt a hand of cards at birth called our genetic code. One of the biggest breakthroughs in science over the last couple of decades is that it's not just about your genes. It's the environment that you create around your genes that matters. In other words, your lifestyle is more important and what you eat every day has a huge impact.

It's my clients who inspired me to write this book, *Cool the Fire: Curb Inflammation and Balance Hormones*. Most of my work has been with midlife and older females to help them lose weight. What I found as I worked with them was that profound inflammation, digestive issues and hormonal imbalance were at the root of their weight loss resistance. But more importantly it was the reason why they felt lousy, couldn't live the life they wanted and, in some cases, even looked and felt 10 years older than they should have.

The purpose of this book is to help you easily make changes that will improve your health and your symptoms. Before you get started, though, we need to get a sense of what is going on for you. So, the first step is to give you individual feedback on your level of inflammation and hormone imbalance. In Chapter 3, you will get connected to your symptoms. This will give you an idea of your level of imbalance.

The second step will teach you 10 High Impact Nutritional Strategies to Renew Vitality to help you change behaviors to reduce symptoms and help get your vitality back. The third step is to show you how to implement these changes through 4 weeks of Mindful Menus and easy recipes that support greater health.

For the menus and recipe part of the book, I primarily offer gluten free, dairy free and low sugar recipes. I find that most of my client's symptoms profoundly improve when they avoid all three. You will find that this type of eating can be delicious focusing on whole foods, quality ingredients and lots of herbs and flavorings.

At the encouragement of some friends, I did add a small section which includes my favorite recipes that contain dairy for those who can tolerate it. Some of my clients do well with small amounts and you may, too. The good news is that if you do some work on healing your gut you may be able to tolerate dairy in the future.

A well balanced nutrient-dense diet sets the foundation to creating hormone balance and curbing inflammation. None of us deserves to suffer from the symptoms associated with hormone imbalance such as profound fatigue, mood issues, struggles with our weight, hot flashes, night sweats, headaches and more. Nor should we need to worry about the risk of heart disease, diabetes, cancer and many other diseases which are the manifestation of uncontrolled inflammation in our bodies.

Eating a diet to cool the fire does not need to be a penance. You don't have to deprive yourself! In fact, it is better for your long-term success if you don't. Once you get yourself balanced you will find that it is easier to make healthy delicious choices that increase your energy and vitality and hopefully help you to dance all night long, or hike a challenging trail, or whatever is out there that you want to achieve. It is my deep hope that this book helps you to get there.

Love,

Ruth

Part I

Chapter 1
The Challenge

My client CG came to me when she was 50 years old with tears in her eyes because all she had to do was look at food to gain weight. I believed her instead of thinking this was just another middle-aged woman with excuses about her weight. Her other symptoms included digestive issues, seasonal allergies, high cholesterol, anxiety, joint pain, congestion, and skin issues. Also, she had had her gall bladder removed 12 years before we started to work together.

She was devastated because she had been to see an endocrinologist (hormone doctor) earlier in the year who told her that her hormones were completely normal. She knew in her heart that this could not be true! So, I asked her to fill out a comprehensive hormone symptom questionnaire.

Since she had about 40 symptoms checked off and complained of all kinds of symptoms, it was clear to me that CG had definite hormone imbalances and significant inflammation.

She had unbalanced cortisol (the stress hormone), which was both very high and very low. She also had estrogen dominance and estrogen deficiency. I know that sounds contradictory, but it is not. More about that in Chapter 11 - Eat for Hormone Balance.

At the root of her weight loss resistance, was a sluggish thyroid which was a direct result of stress hormones that were out of whack as well as significant gut issues and inflammation.

I knew I needed to get results with her fast, so we started with an elimination diet. It became clear that she had sensitivities to both gluten and dairy which put her immune system into overdrive and was causing her painful gastrointestinal symptoms. Her gut was insulted every time she ate these foods.

Another huge breakthrough in recent science is the role the health of your gut plays in your well-being. Many centuries ago Hippocrates stated that "All disease begins in the gut." When you consider all the research that has been published in the last decade about the health of your gut impacting a huge array of issues ranging from mood to diabetes to heart disease, this insight was amazing.

The interplay between your hormones, the health of your gut, and inflammation is powerful. When you have one imbalance, it creates an overall imbalance in the entire body. When you can fix one, it helps the others to heal.

Within 3 weeks CG had lost 11 pounds and felt like a new woman. We went on to work on healing her gut and supporting her adrenals, sex hormones and thyroid with foods, specific supplements and lifestyle modifications. Her mood improved, her energy returned, she was able to lose more weight, and in her own words "feel like I felt 15 years ago".

It made me reflect on what had happened to me as I hit my mid-fifties. I had been working hard and traveling all over the country for my job. It was stressful but I was able to maintain my exercise program and eat well knowing that if I didn't, I would never be able to keep up. Despite that I started gaining weight. In fact, I gained 15 pounds which was puzzling to me.

But more importantly, I couldn't keep up. I was exhausted, not sleeping well, spending my day off sleeping in a chair and my digestion was a disaster. I couldn't figure out what was wrong with me. Part of me began to think it was just aging. And that maybe I needed to work a little harder on self-acceptance.

This went on for about a year. But I really woke up when my immune system started to go sideways. I have had an iron clad immune system all my life. I am one of these people that gets a cold once a decade. But when I got Acute Asthmatic Bronchitis twice in one year, I knew I was in trouble. My primary care doctor had no idea what was wrong with me.

This may be starting to sound familiar to some of you. I wasn't sure where to turn. But fortunately, my yoga teacher was offering a cleanse program. I felt I was at a point where I had nothing to lose. When I was following the cleanse, I felt fantastic — energetic, no digestive issues. We eliminated all the common culprits that cause food sensitivity and consumed foods and consistency of foods designed to rest my gut. Once I started to add foods back to my diet, it became crystal clear that a good part of my symptoms was due to a gluten sensitivity.

Any food sensitivity results in inflammation and can cause leaky gut which leads to hormone imbalance. It was amazing to me how easily I healed once I removed the substance that was causing all the inflammation in the first place. My digestion improved, my sleep got better, my immune system is back to normal and my energy is back.

But this experience with my health and the health of my clients helped me to recognize there were several epidemics going on. Let's talk about them in Chapter 2.

Chapter 2
Epidemics

There are 3 major epidemics that are impacting the health of Americans: inflammation, hormone imbalance, and poor gut health.

Let's start with inflammation also known as the Secret Killer.

You may have been among the few people who read and understood the profound implications for the cover article of *Time* magazine in February 2004 which exposed the link of inflammation to heart disease, cancer, Alzheimer's and many other diseases. That was more than 15 years ago but I still have clients that are new to my practice who don't understand the relationship and are not clear what to do about it. The challenge is that you can have it and not even know it.

Hardly a week goes by without another research study being published that connects inflammation to another disease or harm to the human body. It is generally agreed as the root cause for most diseases that Americans suffer from and die from.

What is inflammation?

Inflammation is the first line of defense for the immune system. Your immune system is an amazingly complex system that is constantly on alert looking to protect us and to find foreign invaders to destroy. This is a good thing because without that first line of defense none of us would have survived early childhood diseases.

A good example is if you look at what happens when you nick your finger by accident in the kitchen. Your immune system goes to work immediately to help protect you from bacteria and to start the healing process. A day or so later you will notice slight redness and swelling around the cut. This is inflammation as your immune system swings into action healing your finger. Acute inflammation helps us to survive.

It's chronic inflammation that becomes an issue for us. We live in a world where we are bombarded by stress, toxins, and dietary imbalances and deficiencies which our immune system sees as challenges that must be dealt with. Over time in this nonstop world of insults, the immune system gets stuck on all the time. This is further complicated by allergies, physical injuries, food sensitivities, infections and health issues like prediabetes, diabetes and being overweight.

Most people are not aware that inflammation is the underlying cause, thinking that the joint pain, fatigue or digestive issues they are experiencing are just natural to the aging process. They are not. Symptoms of inflammation can impact your health and vitality and quality of life but more importantly, inflammation can take your life!

In Chapter 3 – How to Use this Book you will have the opportunity to complete a questionnaire which will help you determine whether you may have inflammation and how serious it might be.

Hormone Imbalance, the second epidemic

As you can see in CG's experience, hormone imbalance is largely ignored and unrecognized in conventional medicine. Estimates say that 85% of women suffer from hormonal imbalance in their lifetime. This, too, is a silent epidemic. And the more I learn about it the more I see that it is not exclusively a female issue.

What are hormones?

Simply put, hormones are chemical messengers. They travel in your bloodstream to tissues and organs. Hormones are an important way that one part of the body communicates with another part. As I am sure you know, when communication isn't optimal things start to go wrong.

Hormones affect many processes in the body, including growth and development, metabolism, sexual function/reproduction, and mood. When your hormones are off it can make you feel exhausted, achy, grouchy and completely out of sorts. Additionally, hormones that are not in balance can lead to inflammation and issues with the health of your gut. You can read more about that in the next section.

First, let's look at the hormones that are out of control in rampant proportions. These include too much insulin, imbalanced sex hormones, too much cortisol, and not enough thyroid hormone.

Too much insulin does not discriminate between males and females. Right now, approximately 50% of people in America have either prediabetes or diabetes. This is largely due to overconsumption of sugar and refined carbohydrates in the diet as well as inactivity. In fact, this has become a worldwide epidemic with both China and India experiencing a very similar prevalence to ours.

Many of my clients who are well on their way to developing diabetes don't even know it. The sad part is that prediabetes is easily reversible with the right nutrition and exercise program, particularly in the early stages.

It's not just about diabetes, though. When your blood sugars are not well regulated, it can have a dramatic impact on your mood. Does the term "hangry" ever apply to you? What I find incredible is the commercial that touts "You are not yourself when you're hungry" offers the victim a candy bar to correct the situation. Yikes! It's the worst solution. The blood sugar spike created by the candy bar will only make the person hungrier and more irritable and lead to high insulin levels.

The next sweeping problem related to hormones are unbalanced cortisol levels. This is due in large part to unchecked stress levels that many of us suffer from. Cortisol, the stress hormone, is out of control in most of the clients that I work with. You can learn more about this in Chapter 11 - Eat for Hormone Balance. But for now, it is important to realize unbalanced cortisol levels can lead to a cascade of problems with your sex hormones progesterone and estrogen and even low levels of thyroid hormone.

The interplay of hormones and inflammation as we age

Hormone imbalance leads to chronic inflammation. As women start to move into perimenopause, hormonal changes cause weight gain in part around the middle of our bodies. There is plenty of evidence that belly fat increases inflammation throughout the body.

As estrogen levels continue to decline and specific inflammatory chemicals increase this leads to joint pain and other symptoms of inflammation. In addition, aging causes us to create excess cortisol as testosterone and estrogen levels naturally drop. Chronically high cortisol levels take a heavy toll on the body from insulin resistance to reduced immune system function.

Excess cortisol is also associated with a low level of thyroid hormone. As a result, many people have trouble losing weight, have chronic infections, fatigue, and a wide variety of other conditions that may further compound the effects of inflammation. So, you can see, it is a vicious cycle.

You may be starting to wonder how well balanced your hormones are. The good news is that you get to look at this in Chapter 3 – How to Use this Book. Before we go there, let's talk about the role that your gut plays in this vicious cycle.

The third epidemic, an unhealthy gut

New research indicates that your digestive system plays a major role in controlling hormones and inflammation. Some 100 trillion organisms called the microbiome reside in your gut, in your mouth, and on your skin. The microbiome is the genetic material of all the microbes – bacteria, fungi, protozoa and viruses – that live on and inside the human body. This microbiome helps us to digest food, protects our brain, regulates our immune system and ultimately inflammation, protects us against unhealthy bacteria, and helps to balance hormones.

Some researchers say that 90% of all disease can be traced back to the microbiome and the health of your gut. Phew! Lots of heavy lifting there.

If you feel that your hormones could be creating symptoms such as fatigue, mood, weight loss resistance, hot flashes, night sweats and all the aggravating symptom that we associate with hormone imbalance, it's important to know that you won't get far in balancing those errant hormones unless you address the health of your gut.

Chapter 3
How to Get the Most from this Book

This book is designed to support you to make changes that will improve your health, your symptoms and your life. As previously mentioned, the first part will give you individual feedback on your level of inflammation and hormone imbalance. Part II will teach you 10 High Impact Nutritional Strategies to help you to understand the basics of a healthy diet. We all know that "diets" don't work. What does work is teaching the concepts of a healthy diet, proper mindset and specific tools that will facilitate mindfulness.

The third step in Part 3 of the book is to show how to make these changes. Part III of the book contains 4 weeks of Mindful Menu suggestions which are simply guidelines to help you implement what you learn in Part II. Every recipe which you find in the Mindful Menus can be found in this book. Plus, many more! So, you have lots of options. More about that in Notes on the Mindful Menus.

Let's start with individual feedback.

I start off every one of my clients with an evaluation so I thought a self-assessment tool would be helpful for you. We will start by having you check off symptoms that relate to hormone imbalance and inflammation. This will give you an idea of how mild, moderate or severe your symptoms might be.

Feedback can be very valuable when it comes to staying motivated and inspired around any changes you might make in your diet and lifestyle.

Please take a few minutes to complete the following forms. You might want to keep a record of your answers to compare in the future after you've taken some steps towards improvement. Remember, just make a checkmark if you have a specific symptom.

Self-assessment for Hormone Imbalance

Check those items that you are experiencing:

☐ Do you have trouble falling asleep or a second wind that keeps you up late?

☐ Do you experience disrupted sleep?

☐ Do you feel like you're constantly racing from one task to the next?

☐ Do you feel wired yet tired?

- [ ] Are you anxious?
- [ ] Do you have memory lapses or feel distracted, especially in stressful situations?
- [ ] Do you crave sugar?
- [ ] Is your waistline expanding or are you experiencing increased belly fat or muffin top?
- [ ] Are you gaining weight despite eating well and exercising regularly?
- [ ] Do you have high blood pressure or creeping blood sugar?
- [ ] Have you been diagnosed with osteopenia or osteoporosis or "bone loss?"
- [ ] Do you experience shakiness, lightheadedness or irritability between meals?
- [ ] Are you exhausted all the time?
- [ ] Do you use caffeine or sugar to bolster your energy and get you through the day?
- [ ] Do you lose stamina, particularly between 2 and 5 in the afternoon?
- [ ] Do you experience backaches and headaches?
- [ ] Do you have insomnia, especially between 1 and 4 in the morning?
- [ ] Do you struggle to get out of bed in the morning?
- [ ] Do you feel unable to cope with stressful situations?
- [ ] Do you have dry and thin skin?
- [ ] Do you feel lethargic and lack energy?
- [ ] Do you get dizzy when you stand up from lying down?
- [ ] Do you struggle to perform daily tasks?
- [ ] Do you crave salty foods?
- [ ] Do you suffer from headaches or migraines?
- [ ] Do you have mood changes, including anxiety or depression?
- [ ] Have you been diagnosed with fibroids, and/or endometriosis?
- [ ] Do you suffer from PMS, irregular menstrual cycle, and/or heavy bleeding?
- [ ] Do you have fibrocystic breasts?
- [ ] Are you experiencing low sex drive?
- [ ] Have you had issues with fertility?
- [ ] Have you ever had a gall bladder problem?

You are halfway there. Keep going!

- [ ] Are you moody and irritable?
- [ ] Do you feel puffy and bloated?
- [ ] Do you take birth control pills or another hormone replacement?
- [ ] Do you experience breast tenderness?

☐ Do you suffer from adult acne?

☐ Have you had an ovarian cyst?

☐ Do you experience brain fog?

☐ Do you find yourself forgetting names or even walking into a room and forgetting why you are there?

☐ Are you experiencing hot flashes and night sweats?

☐ Do you experience vaginal dryness?

☐ Do you feel dry elsewhere — skin, eyes, hair, etc.?

☐ Are you experiencing rapid heartbeat or palpitations?

☐ Do you have thinning hair?

☐ Are you experiencing unwanted hair growth?

☐ Do you have pelvic pain?

☐ Do you have discoloration of arm pits?

☐ Do you have dry skin and/or hair?

☐ Have you experienced hair loss including the outer third of your eyebrow?

☐ Do you have, or have you had high cholesterol?

☐ Do you feel a tingling in your arms?

☐ Are you sensitive to cold?

☐ Do you have cold hands and feet?

☐ Are you exhausted or very fatigued particularly in the morning?

☐ Do you have muscle or joint pain or poor muscle tone?

☐ Do you urinate often?

☐ Are you always thirsty?

☐ Is it difficult for you to lose weight?

☐ Does eating make you feel exhausted and in need of a nap?

☐ Do you have difficulty concentrating?

1 to 5 checks	You likely have a **mild** hormone imbalance
5 to 15 checks	You likely have a **moderate** hormone imbalance
15+ checks	You likely have a **severe** hormone imbalance

Self-assessment for Inflammation

Check those items that you are experiencing:

☐ Do you struggle with your weight even though you know that you are exercising and eating right?

☐ Do you experience gastro-intestinal symptoms such as gas, bloating, belching, constipation, diarrhea or reflux?

☐ Do you experience emotional symptoms such as mood swings, anxiety, nervousness, fear, depression, anger or irritability?

☐ Are you regularly or often fatigued?

☐ Do you experience loss of focus or memory loss that feels like "brain fog?"

☐ Do you have challenges falling asleep or staying asleep?

☐ Have you ever felt that you have reacted to foods such as gluten, dairy or soy?

☐ Do you often catch whatever virus is making the rounds around your office or home?

☐ Do you suffer from joint pain?

☐ Do you experience skin issues such as eczema and psoriasis?

☐ Are you exhausted in the morning but wired at night?

☐ Have you ever been told by a health care professional that you are inflamed?

☐ Have you ever had blood tests with an elevated fasting blood glucose, high sensitivity, CRP, sedimentation rate, homocysteine or ferritin?

☐ Do you experience high levels of stress in your life?

☐ Do you experience headaches on a regular basis?

1 to 3 checks	You likely have **mild** inflammation
3 to 5 checks	You likely have a **moderate chronic** inflammation
5+ checks	You likely have **severe chronic** inflammation

Surprised? And maybe a little disturbed? Try not to put your energy there. The good news is that you can change it. Now you have some great feedback on the level of commitment you might need to improve your hormones, curb inflammation and improve the health of your gut.

The next step is to learn more about the **10 High Impact Nutritional Strategies to Renew Vitality** that are specifically aimed at helping you to renewed vitality. Each one of these concepts was taken into consideration and utilized in the development of the meal plans and recipes.

If you are feeling totally exhausted, fogged in, moody and not ready to dive into the next 10 chapters for the details on these strategies, you may want to dive right into the meal plans! That is perfect and you may find by the second week or so that you feel like circling back around to read about why you are eating these foods.

Part II

10 High Impact Nutritional Strategies to Renew Vitality

1. Be Alert to Food Sensitivities
2. Eat Close to Nature
3. Break Up with Sugar
4. Power Up with Protein
5. Get Your Fiber Fix
6. Focus on Healthy Fat
7. Fight Inflammation with Food
8. Eat for Hormone Balance
9. Improve Your Gut Health
10. Limit Stimulants

Chapter 4
Be Alert to Food Sensitivities

Food is medicine and eating specific healthy foods to support you is one of the best ways to heal the symptoms you may be suffering from. Another good choice is to move toward a lifestyle that supports balance by removing some foods and substances from your daily life.

On the positive side, these 10 High Impact Nutritional Strategies can have a profound impact on how you look and feel. In addition, these guidelines have been used as a litmus test for each of the recipes included in this book.

The #1 Strategy: Be Alert to Food Sensitivities

This is the first and for me the most important strategy. Food sensitivities are a major cause of hormone imbalance and inflammation. It is estimated that as many as 70% of us suffer from some form of food related sensitivity.

A food sensitivity occurs when a person has difficulty digesting a food. Unlike food allergies, these reactions can be delayed and are rarely life-threatening. One of the defining characteristics of a food sensitivity is that a reaction to a food can take up to 72 hours. That is 3 days which is one of the reasons why sensitivities are often hard to identify. When someone experiences joint pain, brain fog or headaches it is typical to think about what you had to eat today or maybe even yesterday but hardly anyone considers that a food eaten 3 days ago could be the culprit.

The important thing to know is that the prevalence of sensitivities is on the rise. Even though they are not as dramatic as allergies, food sensitivities can make us sick. This can lead to obvious symptoms such as intestinal gas, abdominal pain, constipation or diarrhea. But less well-known symptoms include exhaustion, joint pain, headaches, sleep disturbances, congestion, brain fog, mood, and skin issues.

You may wonder how sensitivities can cause such a widespread response in the body. To understand it is important to know a bit about how your GI system works and what happens when you consume a sensitivity food. Every time you eat the food it is an insult to your gut. In the modern world we live in, our gut is already insulted by toxins, including GMO foods and the stress we are exposed to not to mention the times when we can't or don't eat healthfully.

One of the major roles of our GI tract is to keep the outside world out. Think about it this way. Our GI tract is like a long hose that starts in our mouth and comes out the other end. It may be hard to imagine but the length of our gut if you stretched it out is the length of a tennis court. Despite this very important job of providing a barrier to the outside world, the wall of the GI tract is only one cell thick. You can imagine how fragile it is. So, if you are eating foods you are sensitive to instead of maintaining tight juncture between the cells to keep the gut healthy, small tears begin to form in the intestinal wall.

The good news is that your gut can heal these small tears but if you keep eating the foods repeatedly with the usual stress, toxins and processed food layered on top, your gut's restorative powers can't keep up and eventually your gut becomes more like cheesecloth. No longer can it perform its job of keeping the outside world at bay. Instead your body starts to absorb substances that are not intended to pass the gut barrier. These substances are seen as foreign objects.

Your immune system is constantly on alert and ready to remove foreign bodies. Once you start to absorb these foreign bodies your immune system goes into action. Its first line of attack is to dramatically increase inflammation to rid the body of these invaders. This causes systemic inflammation or body-wide symptoms.

Wheat and dairy are considered the most powerful culprits but other substances such as corn, soy, shellfish, food additives like sulfites and artificial colors, and even eggs can cause a sensitivity. If you suspect that you have a food sensitivity it makes sense to eliminate these foods for 3 weeks to see if your symptoms improve. This can be a daunting process and it would be worthwhile to work with a health professional who understands sensitivities.

If you feel that your hormones could be creating symptoms such as fatigue, mood, weight loss resistance, hot flashes, night sweats, and all the aggravating symptoms that we associate with hormone imbalance, it's important to know that you won't get far in balancing those errant hormones unless you address the health of your gut.

This means addressing the health of your microbiome. Did you know that your microbiome is considered an organ? And, that it is more powerful than all your hormone glands put together. More on this in the Chapter 12 – Improve Your Gut Health.

Chapter 5
Eat Close to Nature

Choosing whole foods is one of the best ways to make sure you are getting plenty of fiber and nutrients. Whole foods are foods that have been minimally processed or refined as little as possible and are free from additives, toxins, sugar or other artificial substances. Eating whole foods also means minimizing processed and prepackaged foods.

I urge my clients to think about eating foods that come directly from nature. This means they could be literally plucked from the ground or picked from a tree, shrub or plant or from animals that have been humanely farmed. This includes fruits, veggies, clean protein such as grass-fed beef and lamb, free range poultry and eggs, wild fish, whole grains, and healthy fats such as avocados as well as nuts and seeds.

So, here is a question for you. Is bread considered a processed food? Well, yes according to this definition. So are ready-to-eat cereals, pastas, and crackers. Even if these foods are made from whole grains, they still undergo quite a bit of processing. My recommendation would be to eat the grain whole such as bulgur in a salad or quinoa in a casserole as much as you can.

The more a food is processed the greater the loss of nutrients including fiber. Plainly and simply, we eat too many processed foods in our culture. The best way to assure that you are avoiding processed food is to shop the periphery of the grocery store. Spend most of your time in the produce department and keep out of the aisles where all the foods that contain unpronounceable ingredients reside.

Fruits and Vegetables

The more you focus on eating vegetables and fruits — a minimum of 9 servings per day — the less inflamed you will be which also helps to balance your hormones. Make it a strategy to include fruits and vegetables in every meal. It's not the first time you have heard this, and it won't be the last! This is the one area where scientists and health practitioners from all over the world agree.

Nine servings is not that hard to do. Bear in mind that one serving of veggies is equivalent to ½ cup cooked and 1 cup raw. Fruit servings can vary according to water and sugar content. A good measure for fruit is about ½ cup as a serving. ½ cup of food is just not that much. It is less than half the size of your fist! Nine servings per day is totally doable.

Choose lots of deeply colorful fruits and vegetables every day starting with breakfast. Yes, breakfast! It's not that hard to throw a handful of spinach and some blueberries into a smoothie made with plant milk or some berries on oatmeal, or to cook up some eggs along with some sautéed greens. This is a great way to start your day!

It's also easy to boost your lunch nutritionally by adding vegetables like onion, lettuce, avocado and tomato to your sandwiches. Even better, use a leafy green as a substitute for bread. Soups and salads are an easy choice and a great way to get lots of veggies. At the dinner meal, it is easy to up the vegetable ante. Look at your plate and cover half of it with vegetables! Simple, right?

The easiest way to implement this habit is to think about how you can add color to your meals. And the most nutritious fruits and vegetables are deeply colored through and through. So, think beets, carrots, winter squash, green leafy vegetables, oranges, purple cauliflower, and apricots instead of cucumbers, zucchini, and apples. There is nothing wrong with less color dense foods, you just get a bigger bang for your nutritional buck with deeply colored fruits and veggies.

Cruciferous or brassica veggies are an excellent choice. Vegetables such as cauliflower, broccoli, cabbage, kale and other leafy greens, Brussels sprouts, arugula, turnip, radishes, kohlrabi, watercress, and Bok choy fall into this category. The origin of the name comes from the shape of the flower of the vegetables whose four petals resemble a cross. Cruciferae is Latin for cross bearing.

As a group, these vegetables are simply superstars. You can't find another vegetable group that is as high in vitamin A carotenoids, vitamin C, folic acid, phytonutrients and fiber as the cruciferous vegetables. They are a great source of antioxidant nutrition which is one of the reasons why these veggies are protective against cancer.

Vitamin K is a nutrient that helps regulate our inflammatory response, including chronic, excessive inflammatory responses that can increase our risk of certain cancers. Some researchers suspect that the amazing K content of cruciferous vegetables is related to additional cancer-preventive properties through mechanisms involving better control of inflammation.

In addition, 100 calories' worth of cruciferous vegetables provides us with somewhere between one-third and one-half of a gram of omega-3 fat. Omega-3 fats also offer substantial anti-inflammatory effects.

We have an abundance of fresh crucifers to choose from in the grocery store all year long. Do your best to eat them regularly. Just keep it simple and focus on adding these veggies whenever you can to your meals.

10 Simple Ways to Eat More Cruciferous Veggies

1. Add arugula and watercress to your salads.
2. Chop cauliflower into tiny pieces to create "cauliflower rice" and lightly sauté.
3. Try adding shredded kohlrabi to your coleslaw.
4. Serve fresh radishes with hummus or veggie dip.
5. Roast Brussels sprouts with olive oil, garlic, shallots and walnuts.
6. Stir-fry Bok choy with garlic, ginger and soy sauce.
7. Sprinkle fresh lemon juice and sesame seeds over lightly steamed broccoli.

8. Use cabbage leaves to wrap your next taco or burrito.
9. Add shredded cabbage to sandwiches as a change from lettuce.
10. Add chopped broccoli to omelets and frittatas.

Grains and legumes

Other plant foods include grains, beans and legumes. I like gluten free grains such as quinoa, brown rice, wild rice, millet, amaranth and buckwheat. It depends on your specific hormone imbalance, but for many, it's smart to avoid gluten in your diet.

Grains and legumes overall have become controversial with the advent of paleo eating, the Whole 30 diet, the ketogenic diet, and the autoimmune paleo diet. If you are struggling with an autoimmune challenge such as Hashimoto's, or high levels of inflammation, or diabetes, you may benefit from restricting these foods. But bear in mind these foods are nutrient dense and avoiding them makes it more challenging for you to get a balanced diet. I would recommend that you work individually with a qualified Registered Dietitian or Functional Nutritionist to assure you are getting adequate nutrition.

Nuts and seeds

Nuts and seeds are loaded with fiber and contain some hard-to-find nutrients. They are great additions to recipes to improve flavor and increase nutrients. For example, adding a handful of pumpkin seeds to a salad increases crunch, flavor and just as importantly, magnesium, protein, manganese and iron.

Whole Foods Assure Nutrient Density

The more nutrition that you provide to your body, the better it will function. Did you know that there are thousands of biochemical reactions happening in your body every day? Vitamins and minerals provide the cofactors to make those reactions go in the right direction. In other words, if the nutrient isn't there, the reaction doesn't occur. Magnesium alone is involved in over 300 reactions in your body.

Nutrients are essential for hormone health, to quell inflammation and balance your digestive health. We need them for hormone production, to support our liver where hormones get metabolized and excreted, as antioxidants to reduce toxicity and inflammation as well as for healing our gut.

You will find some great recipes in this book that are designed to support your healing process. The ingredients are based on whole foods to assure nutrient density. And I think you will find that a whole foods diet can be delicious without spending hours and hours in the kitchen. The recipes are designed to be quick, simple and great tasting.

Eat local, seasonal and organic

One of the most important reasons to eat local and seasonal is the health benefits. Seasonal foods are picked at the peak of freshness and offer a high nutritional content. They are chock full of vitamins, minerals, phytonutrients, enzymes and antioxidants that are important for optimal health.

Foods that are not local are harvested early to help the food endure long distance shipping. They don't have the full complement of nutrients they might have had if allowed to ripen naturally. Studies have shown that produce loses nutrients each day after it has been harvested and after three days it has lost 40 percent of its nutritional value.

Unfortunately, produce is often genetically engineered to facilitate packaging for these long trips. Transporting fruit and veggies can also expose them to irradiation to kill germs or preservatives like wax to protect the food during the trip while it is under refrigeration.

Eating local and in season is better for your wallet, too. It's simple supply and demand. For example, think about the basil that is available to us during the winter months. We can spend as much as $5 or more on a puny container of limp and sometimes moldy basil from South America in January. Compare that to the fresh, vibrant, aromatic and over the top bunch you can get from a local farm stand or farmer's market in the summer that costs $2 to $3 at most.

Eating seasonally helps to support our body's cleansing and healing abilities. During the spring, vegetables like dandelion greens, spring onions and garlic greens are great for detoxing your body after a long winter. In the winter, hearty foods like squash and root vegetables are grounding and warming.

Making organic choices, is a key choice in reducing your toxic burden. Each of us is exposed to toxins everyday which makes us more toxic. Choosing organic can make a profound difference in that toxic load. Look at it this way. Our bodies are like big collection containers. The more exposure we have to toxins the more build up occurs until our containers are overflowing. This puts stress on our immune system and liver and creates increased inflammation.

I know going 100% organic can be expensive. I encourage you to check out the Dirty Dozen which is a list of the fruits and vegetable with the highest pesticide and herbicide count according to the Environmental Working Group and the Clean Fifteen which outlines produce that have reduced amounts. Check it out here: www.ewg.org.

Finally, organic, local and seasonal food just hands down tastes better. Generally, what affects nutrients also affects flavor. Food that travels a long way from its origin loses its essence every step of the way. And when it is picked early before it is ripe, the food never gets a chance to develop its full flavor potential. Just compare those flavorless pulpy tomatoes that are available in the grocery store throughout the late fall, winter and spring, to that warm fully ripe delicious tomato from your garden or the farmers market—there is a big difference. Food grown in your local community is usually picked within the last day or two. It's crisp, sweet and loaded with flavor.

Chapter 6
Break Up with Sugar

If you have been struggling with your hormones you may have already concluded that sugar is not your friend. Sugar and refined carbs have a major impact on your hormones. They increase your cortisol, insulin and estrogen levels. One of the best things you can do for your health, cravings and your hormones is to stop eating sugar. But it is not just sugar that we need to be careful about. Refined carbs are a challenge, too.

Refined carbs are foods that have been processed to remove fiber and nutrients like white flour, white rice, white pasta and highly processed ready to eat cereals. Consuming these white foods is just like eating directly out of the sugar bowl.

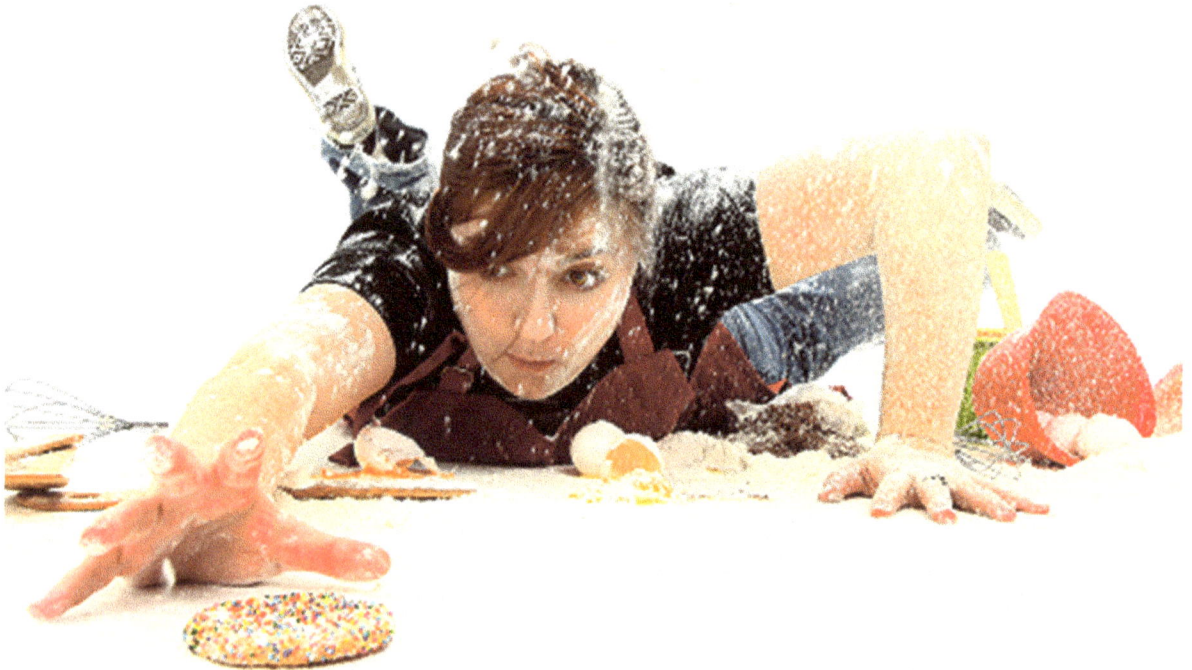

Here's why. The enzymes in our mouths start to break down these foods instantly to sugar. By the time that pasta gets to your intestine where it is absorbed, it is 100% sugar. The sugar then gets absorbed into our blood stream which is where things start to go sideways.

Sugar and its effect on hormones

It is a well-established fact that when we consume carbohydrates, it causes the hormone insulin to be secreted. Insulin plays a vital role in getting sugar in the blood into the cell where it can be used as energy. In fact, insulin is the key which opens the door to let blood sugar into the cell.

The challenge occurs when our diets are high in sugar and refined carbs which causes insulin to be secreted, repeatedly. Eventually, the body becomes insensitive to insulin which is known as insulin resistance. As your cells get insensitive to insulin, it's like the key doesn't fit in the door to the cell any longer. If the door doesn't open, sugar remains in the blood.

As a result, your blood sugar starts to climb, causing more inefficient insulin to be secreted. This puts you at greater risk for prediabetes. It also makes you fatter because insulin is the fat-building hormone. If there is energy being produced and insulin is present, its job is to shunt that energy into your fat cells! Once your insulin starts to climb it causes a vicious cycle. It is a precursor to diabetes. The more carbs, the more insulin resistance, the higher production of insulin which increases the struggle with weight and the greater the risk of diabetes.

Insulin Resistance and Inflammation

Insulin resistance mostly occurs in individuals who are overweight, particularly in people who carry excess weight around their middle. Those excess pounds around the waist set off a series of events which create cytokines leading to chronic inflammation.

Inflammation is the major root cause of most of the chronic diseases that we suffer from in Western society such as heart disease, diabetes, cancer, Alzheimer's and autoimmune diseases. Sugar is one of the most toxic foods that we eat because of its link to inflammation.

What about other hormone imbalances with sugar?

Robert H. Lustig, M.D., Professor of Pediatrics in the Division of Endocrinology at University of California, San Francisco argues that sugar is harmful in significant amounts. It's not just because it's high in calories but because it triggers a toxic chain of reactions in the body that produces harmful fats, hormones, and other metabolic byproducts.

Insulin resistance can also wreak havoc on the ratio of progesterone to estrogen. When these hormones are in balance, we feel happy and calm. When they are out of balance, we feel irritable, anxious, suffer from insomnia, and much more. As women move into menopause, symptoms can get worse and may also include hot flashes and night sweats.

Sugar is Addictive

Some researchers say that sugar is 8 times more addictive than cocaine. In a study conducted at Harvard, investigators fed participants high and low sugar smoothies followed by brain scans. When subjects consumed the high sugar smoothie, the scans of their addiction centers lit up like Christmas trees.

The key player in the reward system of our brain is dopamine. Dopamine receptors are all over our brain. Sugar causes a surge in our dopamine levels and the brain likes that. It seeks that reward repeatedly. The problem is that more and more sugar is required to keep the brain happy.

Just as important is the fact that sugar is very seductive. It is associated with celebration, love and everything that feels nurturing. When we celebrate an achievement or a special day, we don't generally go out for a salad. We want sugar!

The best strategy for sugar management

Get it out of your diet. You will notice that within 7 to 10 days you don't crave it in the same way. I am not saying that you should never eat sugar again. I am just saying that there are some powerful influences at work when it comes to sugar. Be mindful and make sure you have a strategy and plan in place.

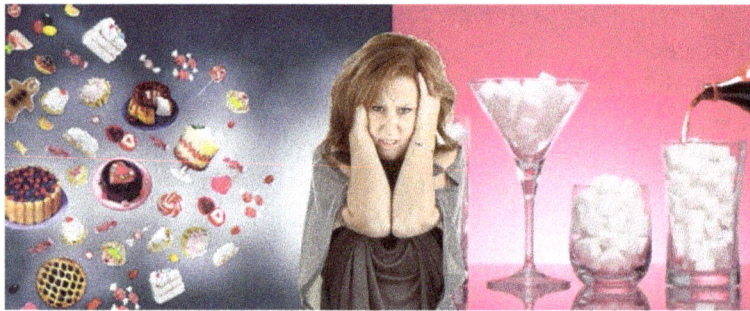

Let's say you are celebrating your anniversary at your favorite restaurant. You know the flour-less chocolate cake there is luscious, and you make a proactive decision to indulge. Just realize that sugar is addictive and the next day your craving for sugar and refined carbs will be powerful. If you have a plan for the next day to eat regular meals and snacks of whole unprocessed foods with plenty of fiber, healthy fat and protein, you will be the one in control not the sugar.

Chapter 7
Power Up with Protein

Protein — not too little and not too much

Consuming an adequate amount of protein is extremely important to your health and your hormones. However, too much protein, especially from animal sources, can increase inflammation in your body and wreak havoc with your health causing symptoms such as joint pain, brain fog, fatigue, redness, swollen joints, skin issues, etc.

What does protein do in the body?

Dietary protein provides essential amino acids (building blocks) that your body can't make on its own and needs to be consumed every day in order to maintain muscle, bone and skin health.

Protein has many critical roles in the body. It does most of the work required in the cell and provides structure, function and regulation of the body's tissues and organs. Proteins are involved in your immune system, digestion, hormones, building of tissue, and repair as well as transport of molecules within the cell and around the body. This nutrient does lots of heavy lifting.

Dietary protein also influences the release of hormones that control appetite and food intake. More about that later.

How much protein do you need?

The right amount of protein for any one individual depends on many factors, including their activity level, age, muscle mass, physique goals and current state of health.

According to the National Academy of Science, the average recommended daily amount of protein for sedentary women is 46 grams and, for sedentary men, 56 grams. You may need more depending on your weight. If you are sedentary, the best formula to determine what you need is 0.8 grams of protein per kilogram of body weight.

To figure out how many kilograms you weigh, simply divide your weight by 2.2. OK, I know this is boring but focus on it because it is important. But if you can't focus right now, go to the meal plans and recipes. Start following the plan. It will help you get better clarity.

Back to the calculation. For example, if you weigh 150 pounds and divide by 2.2, your weight in kgs is 68. Multiply 68 by .8 to get your protein requirements of 54 grams. If you weigh 150, are sedentary and consume more than about 50 grams of protein you are tending toward a high protein diet instead of moderate protein and this can be inflammatory.

If you are highly active, such as an athlete or body builder, you may need more like 1.2 to 2.0 g of protein per kilogram of body weight. In addition, individuals over the age of 65 require somewhere between 1.0 and 1.5 g of protein per kilogram. And of course, if you are pregnant or nursing you also have higher protein needs.

What does that mean in terms of food?

My standard recommendation for protein intake is 20 to 30 grams in each meal for the average person who is sedentary. This breaks down to about 7 to 8 ounces of protein from animal protein in a day or 2 to 3 ounces per meal. If you are consuming vegetable protein you will need at least 2 cups of legumes, 2 cups of high protein grain such as quinoa, and several tablespoons of nuts and seeds in a day.

The healthiest approach in my mind is a combination of both animal and vegetable protein in a day. This way you get lots of variety and better nutrient density. If you are highly active or over the age of 65 you may need one and a half to twice this amount. Bear in mind, everyone is different.

Protein, hormones and appetite control

Protein is the single most important nutrient for weight loss. Eating a high protein breakfast will help you to lose weight and belly fat. The body needs more calories to metabolize protein than for carbohydrate or fat. Protein also provides good satiety value, so you feel full for longer because it activates the body's signals that curb appetite, which reduces cravings and overeating.

This doesn't give you free license to eat as much protein as you want. Pay attention to the guidelines laid out above.

Although studies have shown that protein plays a key role in decreasing belly fat, too much of a good thing will lead to inflammation.

If you are having a challenge bypassing sugar laden snacks like donuts and pastries or even bagels in the morning, try a high protein breakfast instead.

How Much Daily Protein Do You Need?

Take your weight in pounds and divide by 2.2 = your weight in kilograms (kgs.).
Multiply weight in kgs. by 0.8 = your need for protein in grams.

For example, 150 lbs. = 68 kgs.
Avg. Protein need = 0.8 x 68 = 54 g

Highly Active may need 81-136 g
Over 65 may need 68-102 g

A great goal for breakfast protein is to shoot for about 20 grams. Here are some breakfast ideas to help you get there:

❖ Scrambled eggs with veggies (if you tolerate eggs)
❖ Protein Smoothie
❖ Omelet with veggies and sliced avocado on the side
❖ Cottage Cheese and berries (if you tolerate dairy)
❖ Greek yogurt with berries (if you tolerate dairy)
❖ Veggie frittata

Eating protein triggers the hormones that help to control hunger. Research has shown that eating protein decreases levels of the "hunger hormone" ghrelin and stimulates the production of hormones that help you feel full. Women who consumed a diet containing 30% protein reported greater feelings of fullness than when they ate a diet containing 10% protein. If you aim for about 20 to 30 grams of protein per meal you will notice that you feel full for longer and that cravings are in much better control.

The Quality of the Protein you Eat Matters

This is particularly true if you are having challenges with your hormones, specifically estrogen dominance. See Chapter 11 on Eat for Hormone Balance for more on this. The bottom line is that we need to be fully conscious of where our food comes from. The more we can move away from animal sources of protein that contain hormones and antibiotics, the better it is for our hormones. Conventionally farmed foods are higher in antibiotics and hormones. A little well-known fact is that agricultural use of antibiotics is profoundly higher than medical use!

Conventionally farmed animals are also very high in omega-6 fatty acids which are highly inflammatory while organically grown, grass-fed and pasture-raised animals are higher in omega-3 fats which are anti-inflammatory.

CLEAN SOURCES OF PROTEIN

❖ **Pea protein**—contains all 9 essential amino acids so it is a complete protein
❖ **Lentils and other legumes**—lots of fiber and very little fat but some people don't tolerate well
❖ **Seeds**—especially chia, flax, sunflower and pumpkin
❖ **Hemp protein**--one of the most digestible if you have digestive issues
❖ **Nuts**—all kinds
❖ **Cottage cheese and yogurt**—look for hormone and antibiotic free
❖ **Wild caught fish**—especially salmon, herring, sardines and mackerel
❖ **Shellfish**—wild caught
❖ **Poultry and eggs**--Pasture raised
❖ **Red meat**—grass fed

Chapter 8
Get Your Fiber Fix

We already talked a bit about processed food and loss of nutrients, but one of the biggest nutrients of concern is fiber. Fiber which really isn't even considered a nutrient (totally amazing to me) is one of the most important things we eat when it comes to a healthy gut, hormone balance, and good blood sugar control.

What is fiber?

Fiber is simply a carbohydrate found in plant foods. But unlike other carbs, fiber is not easily digested. As a result, it interferes with digestion which helps to slow the absorption of sugar into the bloodstream. This leads to better regulation of your insulin which makes your body less likely to store fat.

This is an important point if you experience weight loss resistance. When your insulin is not well regulated, also known as insulin resistance, the calories you consume are more likely to be converted to fat instead of energy. Here's why. Insulin acts as the key to help sugar get into the cell where it is processed into energy. When you are insulin resistant, the key doesn't work well. The sugar doesn't get into the cell and the calories get stored as energy. This also increases the sugar in the blood which increases insulin resistance and inflammation in your body. This is a vicious cycle! And it is no wonder that you may be struggling with your weight, fatigue and feeling hungry even if you are watching your calories.

This is one of the reasons why foods like refined bread and pasta can be so challenging. Most of the nutrient-dense part of the food has been removed and what remains is quickly absorbed high-carb empty calories. These foods are digested and absorbed quickly which leads to a surge in blood sugar which impacts your appetite and your insulin levels.

Other reasons why fiber is important

Fiber is also important to the health of your gut. If your gut isn't healthy, it's challenging to lose weight. Most everyone knows that fiber is important in keeping us regular. But what most people don't know is that constipation slows weight loss because it creates an unhealthy gut. And if you are "dieting," the lack of fiber only compounds the problem by making you even more constipated.

Fiber has an essential role in keeping your hormones well-balanced. It helps your body to eliminate excess estrogen, a situation known as estrogen dominance. Estrogen dominance has been linked to weight issues because too much estrogen can interfere with your thyroid. Estrogen has an anti-thyroid effect. When dominant it causes thyroid hormone receptors to be less receptive and interferes with the conversion of thyroid hormone from its storage form (T4) to the active form (T3). For more information on estrogen dominance check out Chapter 11 – Eat for Hormone Balance.

Fiber is also essential to the health of your digestive system. It has a profoundly positive impact on the health of your gut bacteria. More about that in Chapter 12 – Improve Your Gut Health.

How much fiber do we need?

The recommended amount of fiber for daily consumption is around 30 to 40 grams. Most Americans consume around 12 to 15 grams per day so you can see we have quite a long way to go to get adequate amounts.

But don't try to solve this problem overnight. Too much fiber too quickly can cause gas and bloating. As you are increasing your fiber intake, make sure you are getting plenty of water. Fiber is like a sponge, so it needs plenty of water. Try to drink about half your weight in ounces. If you weigh 130 pounds, drink around 65 ounces of water per day. If you don't heed this advice, you could end up with the exact opposite of what you are trying to create – constipation. My blog post, *Conquer Cravings by Hydrating* at www.smartnutritionblog.com has some additional information about the importance of proper hydration and how it can also help conquer cravings.

TOP 10 FIBER FOODS

1. **Split peas and other peas and beans**, particularly lentils, black beans and lima beans
2. **Artichokes**
3. **Oat bran**
4. **Berries**
5. **Whole grains** like brown rice, quinoa, wild rice, millet and amaranth
6. **Dark green leafy vegetables**
7. **Oatmeal**
8. **Peas**
9. **Avocados**
10. **Fruits**, especially with skins and seeds, like berries, apples, peaches, pears and plums as well as dried fruits (very small amounts of dried fruit due to the sugar content)

With a few simple and tasty substitutions and additions you can increase your fiber intake in no time flat.

- ❖ Add nuts and seeds to salads, soups, smoothies and veggies.
- ❖ Try doubling or tripling the veggies in a recipe.
- ❖ Add beans to an entrée salad instead of animal protein.
- ❖ Start your day with a good serving of fiber. Choose cereals that contain at least 5 grams or a protein smoothie with added chia or ground flax seeds.
- ❖ Enjoy great high fiber snacks such as hummus and veggies, fresh fruit and nuts, almond butter and apple slices.
- ❖ Choose gluten free grains such as quinoa, brown rice, wild rice, millet and buckwheat.

When it comes to our hormones, one of the hallmarks of having balance is good blood sugar control. When you blood sugar is out of balance it effects your sex hormones, adrenal glands and your insulin levels. Over time, this leads to inflammation. A healthy dose of fiber daily is very helpful in blood sugar control.

Chapter 9
Focus on Healthy Fat

Healthy fats are vital to creating hormone balance, creating satiety, managing inflammation, and helping your body to manage insulin.

Hormone balance

Let's look first at hormone balance. Fats are the basic building blocks of your cell membranes. Fatty cell membranes surround every single cell and control the right balance of hormones to enter your cell. Healthy cell walls mean healthy hormone balance.

This is particularly true for thyroid hormones. If the thyroid hormone can't get into the cell, it can cause a sluggish thyroid.

Certain fatty acids and cholesterol are needed for your body to create hormones. For example, estrogen, progesterone, and testosterone are all steroid hormones made from cholesterol. If you want well-balanced hormones, eating healthy fat is a must.

Fats fill you up

The wonderful thing about fat is that it has a high satiety value. This means it helps to control cravings and manage your waistline because you feel fuller for longer. When you eat fat, cholecystokinin (CCK) and the gut hormone YY Peptide (PYY) are released. These two hormones control appetite and satiety. Appetite is decreased, hunger is suppressed, and you feel satisfied.

Not only does it affect hormones, but fat contributes to the texture, flavor, and aroma of foods making them tastier and more satisfying. When you add healthy fats to your diet and are mindful about how full you feel, you naturally eat less.

Essential Fatty Acids

Healthy fats are a good source of essential fatty acids which are responsible for many different reactions in the body. These fats are essential because the body doesn't manufacture them, and we need to get them from our food. Because they are foundational building blocks for hormone production, fats are important for weight management. Healthy fats that are high in omega-3 fats are also anti-inflammatory.

It's the Omega-6 fats that are highly inflammatory. With the advent of processed and convenience foods the ratio of Omega-6 to Omega-3 fats in our diet has gone from a healthy ratio of 1:1 to more like 20:1. The typical American diet is high in omega-6 fats found in refined oils such as corn, soybean, safflower, sunflower, canola and vegetable oils as well as conventionally fed animal protein.

It's no wonder that inflammation is rampant in our culture. We need to be eating more omega-3 and omega-9 fats for their anti-inflammatory effect. Inflammation is a major reason why I see midlife women struggling with their weight.

It always surprises me when I hear women in my practice say that they are afraid to eat foods like olives, avocado and nuts because they are high in calories. This is an outdated concept and it's contrary to modern science. We need to let it go. If it is healthy fat, it helps with many aspects of appetite control and metabolism.

Trans fats

On the other hand, eating foods with the wrong kinds of fat will help you to gain weight. Trans fats found in pie crusts, cupcakes, donuts, cookies and other baked goodies are likely to be loaded with partially hydrogenated fat — READ trans fats. Make sure you are reading the ingredients on the label of prepared foods. Or better yet, stay away from processed prepared foods altogether.

Fat keeps your insulin levels healthy

As mentioned earlier, one of the most dangerous hormone epidemics we suffer from is overproduction of insulin. For this reason, the rate of diabetes is growing at an alarming rate around the world. Unfortunately, in the US, one out of every 2 people is significantly headed in the wrong direction when it comes to risk of this excessively debilitating disease.

The good news is that for many people diabetes is reversible. This conversation is outside of the scope of this book and content for another book but following the **10 High Impact Nutritional Strategies to Renew Vitality** can make a major difference. The name of the game is to keep your insulin levels low.

In Chapter 6 – Break Up with Sugar, we reviewed the role that insulin has in blood sugar challenges, weight gain and inflammation. Carbohydrates, particularly sugar and refined carbohydrates cause insulin to climb. Too much protein in our diet can also increase insulin. There are 3 primary sources of energy (calories) for the body to use as fuel: carbohydrates, protein, and fat. We have already learned that carbs and protein can increase insulin but what about fat?

There is some evidence that saturated fats may cause an increase in insulin, but healthy fats do not. Healthy fats will also help suppress your appetite, reduce the calories you eat in a day, support your heart health, and help to boost your metabolism.

Here are some delicious foods with good amounts of healthy fats:

9 HEALTHY FAT FOODS
TO HELP TAME INFLAMMATION

1. **Fatty fish**—One of the best sources of omega-3 fats are fatty fish such as salmon, herring, sardines and mackerel. An added benefit of fish is its short cooking time which allows you to get dinner on the table more quickly.
2. **Chia seeds**—Loaded with amino acids, healthy fatty acids and fiber, chia seeds are a great choice. One of the benefits is how easy they are to use. Just add them to a smoothie, granola, a soup or casserole. Ground flax seeds are great fat too.
3. **Olives and olive oil**—Extra virgin olive oil can add lots of flavor and healthy fat to your meals. A word of caution with olive oil is to avoid heat above 350° F. If you are roasting veggies at 375° F or searing fish, chicken or meat, use a more stable oil like avocado oil. When it comes to olive oil look for real extra-virgin organic cold pressed oil in a darkly tinted bottle. Olives are a great addition to veggies, soups and casseroles because they pack a lot of flavor. More info about olive oil in my blog post *Let's get real…finding real extra-virgin olive oil* at www.smartnutritionblog.com.
4. **Butter**—Grass fed butter is a good source of conjugated linoleic acid (CLA) a fatty acid which is associated with improving lean muscle mass and reducing body fat. It contains butyric acid, a short chain fatty acid with anti-inflammatory properties, omega-3's, and up to 5 times more CLA than butter from grain fed cows.
5. **Pasture raised organic eggs**—These eggs are a great choice because they contain more omega-3 fats than conventionally raised eggs and are lower in cholesterol.
6. **Coconut oil**—Coconut oil contains medium chain triglycerides (MCT's) which have many health benefits. MCT's are easier to digest, not readily stored as fat, available for immediate energy, are anti-fungal and anti-microbial. They are anti-inflammatory which should be helpful in heart disease prevention, but the jury is still out for some scientists. Even though coconut oil increases good cholesterol (HDL), we still don't really know how coconut oil effects heart disease. The recommendation is to use it more sparingly.
7. **Avocados**—This versatile fruit is largely made of oleic acid which is a monounsaturated omega-9 fatty acid with many health benefits. Add avocados to smoothies (makes the texture velvety), salads, use it as a spread on toast, and add it to sandwiches. Or just eat it pure—half an avocado with lemon juice and your favorite seasonings.
8. I also like **avocado oil** for cooking. It is a monounsaturated fat which raises good cholesterol while lowering the bad and it has a high smoke point. This makes it a great choice for higher heat cooking like roasting veggies or searing meats.
9. **Walnuts**—Many nuts and seeds have healthy fats, but walnuts have the most omega-3 fats.

All these foods have been integrated into the **Mindful Meal Plans in Part III** of this book.

Chapter 10
Fight Inflammation with Food

One of the best ways to fight inflammation lies in the kitchen not the medicine chest. Many delicious foods have a profound effect on inflammation in the body.

Mediterranean cooking is one of the best examples of a cuisine that is great for cooling inflammation. Countries to look for inspiration from this cuisine include Italy, Spain, Croatia, France, Greece, Spain, Morocco and Portugal. Not only is the Med Diet great for reducing inflammation and the risk of heart disease, diabetes, cancer and many other diseases, it is rich with fresh flavorful ingredients and not complicated to cook.

The diet is based primarily on fruits and vegetable as the foundation with healthy clean protein (largely as fish), healthy fats, whole grains and legumes, seeds and nuts, and small amounts of dairy

Let's start with vegetables because they are so powerful

Eat the rainbow. This means making sure your plate is as colorful as you can make it. Why? Antioxidants like carotenoids and flavonoids which give fruits and veggies their bright color, can help to reduce your body's inflammatory response. These antioxidants reduce oxidation also known as free radical damage which reduces inflammation.

Use leafy greens and cruciferous vegetables to make stunning salads, garlicky greens, fragrant soups and stews, or oven-roasted medleys. Vegetables are vitally important to the fresh tastes and delicious flavors of a healthy diet.

Broccoli sprouts are a smart veggie to use regularly because they are so easy to add to side dishes, salads, smoothies, soups and casseroles. They are also known to be a lot more powerful than the mighty broccoli and other crucifers. All these veggies are nutritional powerhouses.

Beets fall into the category of vegetables that are deeply colored through and through. In fact, all highly pigmented veggies are a good choice. The deep dark color of beets assures that they are high in inflammation fighting antioxidants. Beets are simple to add to salads and soups, plus they make a great side dish. But many people avoid beets because they seem difficult to work with. And that makes sense to me because I don't love peeling beets either but check out the recipes for beets in the back of the book for any easy way to get past this obstacle.

Another great veggie for inflammation is celery. Celery has both antioxidant and anti-inflammatory properties. It is an excellent source of potassium which plays an important role in getting rid of toxins. Toxins are a source of free radical damage and inflammation. Celery is simple to use in soups, stews and casseroles, and contributes a lot of flavor.

Fruits are a good close second to veggies

Berries are very anti-inflammatory, especially blueberries. Again, it is the deep pigment that is responsible for that antioxidant protection. But other berries are great for you too, such as raspberries, blackberries, and strawberries. But don't forget about goji, acai, bilberries and cranberries. Raspberries and blackberries bring a healthy dose of about 8 grams of fiber to the party.

Another benefit of berries is their low glycemic index. This means any sugar in the fruit is more slowly absorbed which is great for your blood sugar levels and your hormones.

Cherries are a great source of antioxidants too, though they tend to be higher in sugar. This doesn't mean you need to avoid them but that you need to practice good portion control. About 1/2 cup is enough.

Apples help to cool the fire because they are a great source of quercetin. Quercetin is a flavonoid which is an extremely strong antioxidant that is highly anti-inflammatory and fights cancer.

Avocados are classified as fruit and are a delicious fiber-filled source of healthy fats. Olives are a great way to cool the fire and add lots of flavor, too.

Finally, in the fruit family, is pineapple. It is the bromelain which is an enzyme in pineapple that helps with inflammation. This delicious fruit is a great snack and a good dessert food. Just go easy on the portion size because pineapple has a higher glycemic index.

Omega-3 fat containing foods

Other substances found in food such as omega-3 fats are known to be highly anti-inflammatory. As one of the highest sources of omega-3 fats, salmon is a great choice, but mackerel, herring and sardines are good choices too! Research shows that omega-3 fats may help lower the risk for heart disease and arthritis largely due to the inflammation lowering effect.

All kinds of seafood are a good choice. Look for wild fish instead of farmed to reduce your exposure to contaminants and dyes.

Other great sources of omega-3 fats include chia and flax seeds. Chia seeds are tiny packets of super nutrition. They supply a remarkable amount of nutrients in a very small portion—about 2 tablespoons. Despite their tiny size, chia seeds are among the most nutritious foods on the planet. The ancient Aztecs and Mayans valued these little powerhouses for their energy-boosting-properties. Besides having a great omega-3 profile, they are a good source of protein, fiber, antioxidants and minerals.

Flax seeds are another great source of omega-3 fat. They, too, are a great source or fiber which is important for the health of your gut. An unhealthy gut can be a major source of inflammation in the body. More about this in Chapter 12 – Improve Your Gut Health. Flax seeds can also be helpful for specific hormone imbalance. You will learn more about this in Chapter 11 – Eat for Hormone Balance.

Walnuts are the nut with the highest amount of omega-3 fats. You can grab them on the go for a great snack or use them in salads with a healthy drizzle of olive oil or add them to any veggie dish to up the flavor and nutrition. Other nuts fight inflammation, too, so don't neglect them. You can add quite a lot of nutrients to your meals when you add nuts to food preparation.

Switch to Whole Grains

Whole grains are naturally rich in many important nutrients. Their nuttier taste and extra fiber keep you satisfied for hours. If you are sensitive to gluten stick with gluten free whole grains, including brown, black or red rice, wild rice, quinoa, amaranth, millet and buckwheat. If you tolerate gluten, traditional Mediterranean grains like bulgur, barley, and farro are delicious and add good variety. Whole grain pasta is a good choice on occasion.

Make sure you are checking the labels on foods containing grains. There are many grain products on the market that appear to be whole. The closer you look at the label, the more assured you can be that you have made a good choice. The first ingredient on the label should be whole wheat or whole grain. Also, look at the fiber content of the food. If it is less than 3 grams per serving you would be better served with a product that is higher in fiber.

Some individuals have challenges digesting whole grains and other foods. There is a buzz around the internet that whole grains may not be good for your health. The claim is that grains cause flatulence but more importantly are contaminated with dangerous lectins. Some say that eating lectins can cause inflammation and intestinal permeability. Although I do believe that maintaining a healthy gut in the world, we live in today is not easy, to my mind lectins are not the culprit.

Let's look at the lectin conversation because in some nutrition circles, lectins are the enemy. Lectins are a category of proteins that bind to carbohydrates. Plant lectins are found in fruits, vegetables, nuts, grains and legumes. The theory is that they cause inflammation and intestinal permeability, leading to chronic disease.

But many traditional cultures consumed diets that are based on all these foods without the same increase in chronic disease. So, it seems like an intellectual leap to say lectins are the culprit. Grains, legumes and nightshade vegetables have received the most negative press.

It is well known that certain lectins such as ricin (from castor beans) and hemagglutinin from kidney beans are toxic to humans and animals. But it is important to understand that the toxic substance is only a problem in raw kidney beans. And I don't know anyone who eats kidney beans raw, or ricin for that matter. But some people don't cook beans and grains properly and this can lead to small amounts of lectins in our foods.

The important take home here, then, is to make sure you cook beans and grains properly. This is particularly true if you have digestive issues around grains or beans. But that doesn't mean that some folks shouldn't avoid lectins. For people who can't tolerate these foods, it is more likely that they have compromised gut function and may need to heal their gut to have a better tolerance of these foods. This is important because there are many beneficial nutrients, including essential vitamins, minerals, antioxidants, phytochemicals, and fiber found in whole grains, legumes, and other lectin-containing foods.

If you are having digestive issues and are frustrated or puzzled about what may be causing them, my best advice is to work with a Registered Dietitian Nutritionist who is well trained to help you identify the problem and to help you get on a program to relieve your symptoms. These issues are very individual and require customized care.

Legumes

In addition to all the nutrients present in legumes, they are a great source of vegetable protein as well as an excellent source of fiber. It makes sense to try to replace animal protein with some vegetable protein in your diet. A good rule of thumb is to eat at least one to two vegetarian dinners a week. If you use legumes such as lentils, peas and beans in these meals it will help you meet your fiber target and increase variety in your nutrient intake. Legumes are plant food and plant foods are anti-inflammatory.

Healthy Fats

In addition to the benefits outlined in Chapter 9 – Focus on Healthy Fat and the omega-3 fats conversation above, healthy fats are an important mainstay of an anti-inflammatory diet. Choose your oils carefully. Extra-virgin olive oil is rich in the healthy monounsaturated fat, oleic acid. Oleic acid helps to reduce inflammation and may have a beneficial effect on genes that are linked to cancer.

Large amounts of inflammation-fighting antioxidants are found in real extra-virgin olive oil. A key antioxidant known as oleocanthal has been shown to work similarly to ibuprofen, an anti-inflammatory drug. But real olive oil can be hard to find. Read my blog post *Let's get real…finding real extra-virgin olive oil* at www.smartnutritionblog.com for more info. Some of the most well-known olive oil on the grocery shelf is not really genuine olive oil. Also, olive oil is heat sensitive, so it is best used in cold food prep or in recipes where the temperature of the oven or stove top does not exceed 350° F.

Coconut oil can be a good cooking alternative. It's anti-inflammatory, which is great, but it is also saturated fat, so I recommend small portions. Using a bit of coconut oil in cooking is fine but putting 2 or more tablespoons in smoothies might be risky if you are at risk for heart disease. The jury is still out for some scientists. Even though coconut oil has been shown to increase the good cholesterol (HDL), we don't really know how coconut oil affects heart disease. The recommendation is to use it sparingly.

I also like avocado oil for cooking. It is a monounsaturated fat which raises good cholesterol while lowering the bad and it has a high smoke point. This makes it a great choice for higher heat cooking like roasting veggies or searing meats.

Healthy herbs and spices

When we think of herbs and spices, we tend to think of their value as adding flavor to our food. But these culinary delights add a big punch when it comes to nutrients for healing. Many of us are increasingly looking for alternatives to medication. Herbs and spices are good options in many cases.

The two best well-known spices when it comes to fighting inflammation are turmeric and ginger. Curcumin is the primary component of turmeric demonstrating anti-inflammatory activity but there are several other constituents in turmeric that also have an effect. Make sure you consume pepper and a little fat when you are consuming turmeric or the active compound, curcumin. Both make it more absorbable.

Turmeric can be easily added to soups, stew, casseroles, stir fry and veggies dishes. Or fix yourself a delicious Golden Milk Latte. This is especially comforting during the colder months.

The anti-inflammatory power in ginger is off the charts thanks to a compound called xanthine. Fresh, dried or in supplement form, ginger is another immune modulator that helps reduce inflammation caused by overactive immune responses.

Try using a chunk of fresh ginger (about the size of your thumbnail) or a drop of certified pure therapeutic grade ginger essential oil in your smoothies. It makes them delicious and very fresh tasting and reduces inflammation. You can add ginger to sautéed veggies, soups, stews, stir fries and casseroles.

Ginger tea or latte is another great way to enjoy this powerful tool that helps to put out the fire.

Green herbs such as thyme, rosemary and oregano contain powerful antioxidants and are potent tools to cool the fire.

TOP ANTI-INFLAMMATORY HERBS & SPICES

Turmeric	Ginger
Curry powder	Garlic
Cinnamon	Cloves
Black Peppercorns	Cilantro
Nutmeg	Rosemary
Thyme	Oregano
Basil	Chamomile
Celery Seed	Cardamom
Chili peppers	Cayenne pepper

Foods that cause inflammation

Making good anti-inflammatory choices is a great first step toward cooling the fire. But you want to make sure not to negate this positive effect by choosing foods that can cause inflammation.

Here is what you need to **steer clear of:**

Sugar — Sugar is one of the most highly inflammatory substance that we eat. It's addictive and seductive. See Chapter 6 – Break Up with Sugar for more info on how to get this habit under better control.

Refined Carbs — We already talked about refined carbs in Chapter 6 – Break Up with Sugar. Eating these foods is just like eating sugar. Kiss those pastries, cookies, crackers, and so on goodbye. Your body will thank you for it.

Unhealthy fats — Refined oils such as soybean, vegetable, safflower and sunflower oils are highly inflammatory due to their higher content of omega-6 fats. Soy oil is everywhere in processed foods which is one of the reasons why you want to avoid them.

Foods like shortening and baked goods are full of trans fats which is about the unhealthiest fat you can eat. Watch for the words "partially hydrogenated fat" on the label. Some may even be labeled as "0 trans fat" but have only reduced just enough to legally make that claim. Beware.

Conventionally farmed animals — These sources of protein are corn fed which makes them considerably higher in omega-6 fats (inflammatory) than grass-fed or pasture-raised animals.

Fried foods — Most fried foods are made with soy oil and it is impossible to know how frequently the deep fryer fats get changed. As that fat breaks down with reheating it becomes even more inflammatory.

Processed meat — Processed meat (hot dogs, sausage, deli meats) is high in inflammatory compounds like AGEs (advanced glycation end products)

Too much alcohol — Heavy consumption of alcohol may lead to inflammation and could also cause changes to the gut lining resulting in systemic inflammation.

Foods that create sensitivities — Depends on the individual, but wheat, dairy, eggs, corn, soy and eggs are the major culprits.

Consider omega-3 fat and vitamin D supplementation

The omega-3 fatty acids in foods appear to lower the production of inflammatory proteins. Research has shown that a diet high in omega-3 fatty acids may decrease inflammation to the same extent that aspirin and other nonsteroidal anti-inflammatory drugs (NSAIDs) do. As you will read in Chapter 12 – Improve Your Gut Health, NSAIDS have a negative impact on your gut. Omega-3 supplementation may help.

Vitamin D is more like a hormone than a vitamin. In addition to supporting the immune system it plays a major role in the development of strong bones and preventing chronic disease. Its preventative effect is largely because it is a **powerful anti-inflammatory**. Research indicates it may play an important role in the prevention of diabetes, certain cancers, multiple sclerosis and other auto-immune disorders, depression, heart disease, high blood pressure, and stroke.

In addition, some scientist say that vitamin D plays an important role regulating the immune system by helping to shut down the inflammatory response.

Chapter 11
Eat for Hormone Balance

If you scored higher than 10 on the Hormone Imbalance questionnaire (Chapter 3), I am going to guess that your cortisol levels are unbalanced, your progesterone and estrogen may be fighting with one another, your thyroid is at the very least sluggish, and your insulin levels may have started to climb.

That's the bad news. The good news is that you probably don't need to turn to medication to get your energy, waistline or mood back.

As I mentioned before, food is powerful medicine and eating proper foods and practicing good lifestyle habits can often get you back in balance pretty fast.

Let's look at cortisol balance first

In the world of non-stop stimulation and stress we live in, it's easy to create adrenal fatigue. The adrenal glands are walnut sized glands that sit on top of your kidneys. They are responsible for producing many hormones and helping you respond to stress and perceived threats by secreting the hormone cortisol, also known as the stress hormone.

Deadlines, crazy schedules, and never having enough time to do what needs to be done creates an outpouring of cortisol. Eventually, your cortisol levels become elevated which can lead to difficulty falling asleep, disrupted sleep, anxiety, blood sugar irregularities, mood issues, high blood pressure, increased belly fat, and more.

The more demand you put on your adrenal glands to keep up the harder it is for them to deliver. In the long run, the adrenal glands can't keep up with the demand over time and you start to experience low

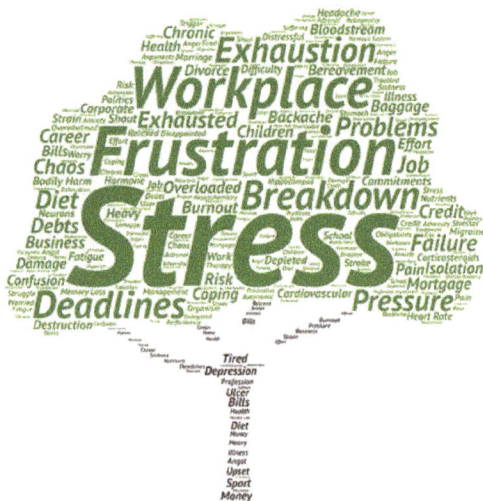

cortisol levels. At this point, you may start to experience burn out, fatigue, loss of stamina, a negative point of view, and crying jags. Your immune system may start to falter, and your GI system will be challenged.

The stress response is innate and tied to our very survival. Back in the caveman days this was a great adaptation. As soon as you saw the saber-toothed tiger cross your path, your body would start to pour out substances that would increase your blood pressure, blood sugar and respirations so you could flee from the danger. In modern times our stressors are not the same. But the brain has not adapted. It perceives any threat as major. Even if it is merely a looming deadline, a schedule conflict, or too much to do with too little time.

Because the adrenals are all about our survival, they tend to get priority for resources to help in hormone production. As a result, the sex hormones and the thyroid gland suffer. Feeling good, when it comes to your hormones, is all about balance. When your adrenal glands start to go sideways, so can everything else.

There is a lot you can do to heal your adrenals when it comes to nutrition and lifestyle which I have outlined in **10 Steps to Heal Your Adrenals**. As you will note, adaptogens can also be useful in supporting your adrenal glands. You may have heard of these herbs before: Ashwagandha, Rhodiola Rosea, Schisandra and Ginseng. These herbs help your body to adapt better to the stress. Maca is also helpful. More about that in the section on Post-menopausal Vitality. You can learn more about these helpful herbs at my blog post: Boost Your Stress Resilience with these Special Herbs (Adaptogens) at www.smartnutritionblog.com.

But one of the hardest lessons a lot of us need to learn is that our crazy busy lifestyle must change. You could follow every nutrition tip and take handfuls of supplements every day but none of it will work if you don't find a way to relax on a regular basis. We live in a society that thinks it is normal for us to experience burnout and exhaustion on a regular basis. In today's fast paced world many of us are overworked, under-rested and it never stops. If you want your hormones to be balanced, find ways to deeply relax regularly.

This requires some soul searching on your part to figure out what really nurtures you. Is it a walk in nature? A well-deserved nap on a regular basis? A quiet weekend away? Or simply 10 to 15 minutes devoted to yourself daily? Only you know what resonates best!

Do your best to follow each of these tips but remember, if you want your hormones to be balanced, be sure to find ways to deeply relax regularly.

If this information feels a little overwhelming. No worries. Just flip ahead to try the Mindful Menus and recipes, especially the hormone balancing smoothies. You can come back later to learn the "why" behind the changes you are making. Following the meal plans makes it easier to feel better fast.

Estrogen Balance is also key

Do you experience puffiness, headaches, weight gain and irritability? In the world we live, it is not uncommon for midlife women to experience estrogen dominance. We are constantly barraged by estrogen from the food we eat, the products we use, and the toxins we are exposed to. Environmental estrogens are everywhere. So, if you are feeling overwhelmed, moody, irritable, suffering from insomnia and struggling with your weight, it may be worthwhile to look at whether your hormones, particularly estrogen and progesterone, are unbalanced.

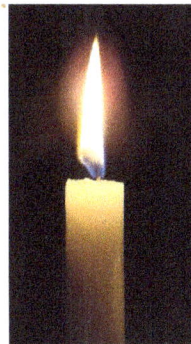

10 STEPS TO HEAL YOUR ADRENALS

1. **Eat regular meals and snacks.** When you go too long without eating, your adrenals go into overdrive. I recommend 3 meals and 2 snacks per day.

2. **Eat breakfast like a king, lunch like a prince, and dinner like a pauper.** This helps support cortisol and maintain hormone balance.

3. **Cycle your carbs.** Try eating a low-carb breakfast, moderate amounts of healthy carbs in the afternoon, and higher amounts of healthy, slow carbs for dinner. The carbs will cause an insulin response which lowers your cortisol. A low carb diet can promote weight loss, but it is not the best choice if your cortisol levels are off.

4. **Avoid sugar** which is easier said than done. It's addictive. It's natural to crave sweets when your blood sugar is low, but the short-term energy from these foods quickly lowers blood sugar making you feel hungry and tired and puts your adrenals into overdrive. See more in Chapter 6 – Break Up with Sugar.

5. **Include protein in your meals and snacks.** This will help to control your blood sugar, your cravings, and your energy levels. See Chapter 4 – Power Up with Protein.

6. **Eat healthy fats.** Fat provides building blocks for healthy hormone production. There are lots of healthy fat choices to help with hormone balance and inflammation.

7. **Avoid foods you are sensitive to and heal your gut.** Coming up next, Chapter 12 – Improve Your Gut Health.

8. **Supplement your diet.** I recommend several essential nutrients to help heal adrenals: vitamin C, a good B complex vitamin, a fish oil supplement, and adaptogens. An effective amount of vitamin C is 250 to 500 mg a day to help replenish cortisol levels. A good recommendation for fish oil is 2000 mg/day. Fish oil lowers cortisol and reduces heart rate and sympathetic nervous system response to stress.

   Herbal adaptogens not only reduce the effect of stress but help to reestablish a healthy cortisol balance. For more info on adaptogens check out my blog post: *Boost Your Stress Resilience with these Special Herbs (Adaptogens)* at www.smartnutritionblog.com

9. **Avoid caffeine and alcohol.** Caffeine can mimic the flight or fight response while alcohol can depress the function of the adrenals.

10. **Relax, relax, relax.** Make it a high priority. No one single thing can heal your adrenals. Diet, supplements, lifestyle modifications and relaxation are key. BUT,

Even if you do all these actions, if you avoid the relaxation piece, it is not likely that your adrenals will recover.

Estrogen is the hormone that gives women their feminine curves, helps control the menstrual cycle, and is important in childbearing. Estrogen also keeps cholesterol in check, protects bone health, and influences your mood.

Progesterone, on the other hand, stimulates and regulates various body functions, like ovulation, and plays a major role in maintaining pregnancy. But it also balances out estrogen with its calming effect.

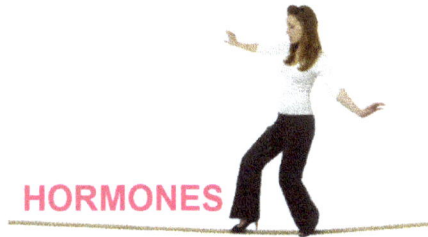

HORMONES

Estrogen dominance occurs when estrogen-progesterone balance is not harmonious and can be responsible for many of the symptoms of perimenopause and menopause.

Signs and symptoms of estrogen dominance

Symptoms of estrogen dominance include bloating and puffiness, history of abnormal pap smears, endometriosis and fibroids, acne, mood swings and irritability, anxiety, migraines, insomnia, breast tenderness or ovarian cysts.

The primary symptom that AR came to see me for was her history of migraines. But she was also concerned about inflammation. She was in her mid-50's and perimenopausal. She felt irritable and was experiencing insomnia, anxiety, hot flashes, and brain fog. She also complained of digestive issues and joint pain. Her evaluation indicated that her cortisol levels were unbalanced, she was estrogen dominant and deficient, and her thyroid was sluggish. She had experienced Lyme several years before and her joints still bothered her.

Since estrogen dominance plays a role in migraines, we put her on a nutrient dense eating plan to support her liver which also minimized estrogen intake and toxins. She also avoided gluten and dairy which helped her joints tremendously. Since her evaluation indicated that her cortisol was out of balance, we started her on herbs to support her adrenals and on a regimen of supplements for estrogen dominance.

Most of my clients suffer some level of magnesium deficiency. AR was no exception. Magnesium can be exceptionally helpful for both sleep and migraines. Within a week, her migraines were gone, and her other symptoms resolved as well.

Estrogen dominance can have a major impact on how you feel every single day. But more importantly, estrogen dominance is thought to be responsible for many types of cancers. Hormone imbalance could be one of the leading causes of breast, uterine, and prostate cancer.

The estrogen and progesterone partnership

Estrogen and progesterone need to be in balance for us to feel well. They are like dance partners, enhancing the action of one another and keeping each other in check. Progesterone keeps estrogen in check.

As women age there is a natural decline in progesterone. This can leave a relative excess of estrogen. Even if you have low levels of estrogen you can have estrogen dominance when progesterone levels are very low.

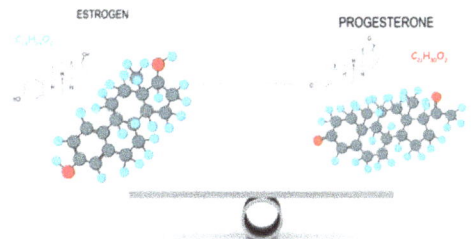

ESTROGEN   PROGESTERONE

Please meet my client, CK. She came to me with digestive issues, anxiety, very heavy periods, irritability, profound fatigue and restless leg syndrome. She was about 50 pounds overweight and she said she was gluten sensitive. Her evaluation indicated high cortisol levels, low progesterone and estrogen dominance and deficiency.

She started an elimination diet where we found that she was sensitive to both gluten and dairy. Then we initiated a supplement regimen aimed at improving both her progesterone and estrogen levels. Because of the food sensitivities her gut needed healing. The primary focus was removing the insulting foods and supporting the function of her gut through a nutrient dense diet and supplements.

She lost 20 pounds. All her symptoms improved, and she remains gluten and dairy free. Since CK has 4 children, she is thrilled to have her life back.

The estrogen dominance/estrogen deficiency syndrome generally occurs in late perimenopause or menopause when even small amounts of estrogen are unchallenged.

In addition to all the symptoms we already reviewed estrogen dominance can also result in a weight struggle. This is because estrogen has an anti-thyroid effect. It causes thyroid hormone receptors to be less receptive and interferes with the conversion of thyroid hormone from its storage form (T4) to the active form (T3).

One of the most powerful things you can do if you are estrogen dominant is to give your liver some love. Since the liver breaks down estrogen, anything that interferes with it like alcohol, excess caffeine, drugs or toxins will decrease its ability to help the body get rid of estrogen. Certain foods such as beets, sprouts, cilantro, cruciferous veggies, greens, and particularly, dandelion are supportive to your liver. Cruciferous veggies are super stars because they help to shift your estrogen metabolism in a positive direction.

Just as important is moving away from conventionally farmed animals. We have already discussed that they are managed using large amounts of hormones and antibiotics. Consuming organic and grass-fed meat will help to keep your estrogen burden lower.

The third high impact behavior that packs a punch when it comes to estrogen is to avoid xenoestrogens. These include pesticides, herbicides, fungicides, plastics, fuels, car exhausts, dry cleaning chemicals, industrial waste, and personal care products that contain phthalates. Xeno stands for "strange" or "alien." Xenoestrogens are a subcategory of the endocrine disruptor group that specifically have estrogen-like effects. Check out Environmental Working Group at www.ewg.org for more information.

Another behavior to improve estrogen-progesterone balance is increasing your ratio of healthy to unhealthy bacteria with fiber. Fiber helps to improve digestion and pulls estrogen out of the body. Great sources of fiber can be reviewed in Chapter 8 – Get Your Fiber Fix.

Postmenopausal Vitality

As we move past menopause, our ovaries start producing less estrogen naturally. But luckily our adrenal glands and our fat stores help to keep us protected. Sometimes it's not enough, though, and we can get symptomatic.

In addition to defining you as a woman, estrogen also builds and maintains the structure of our sex organs and regulates the menstrual cycle. Just as important, it protects our hearts, bones, brains and eyes. Estrogen also helps to keep our cholesterol levels down and plays a role in our longevity. So, this hormone is vital as we go through the aging process.

Some of the most troubling symptoms of low estrogen include weight gain (in all the wrong places!), mood issues such as anxiety and depression, brain fog, loss of memory, fatigue, low libido, dryness, rapid heartbeat, and hot flashes or night sweats. And of course, insomnia.

Here's the challenge: I think we (and the medical community) often confuse low estrogen with the aging process, thinking there is nothing we can do to about it. I don't agree. Managing your food, supplements and lifestyle can go a long way toward helping you with many of these symptoms. Menopause is like our second spring. Let's use every resource we can to stay on top of our game.

Foods that can cause problems:

Gluten — If you are sensitive to it. There is a link in the scientific literature between gluten sensitivity and ovarian reserve where imbalanced estrogen is a common side effect of gluten intolerance. Most of my clients who come to me for weight management start with a 2-week elimination diet which excludes gluten among several other foods that can cause sensitivity and inflammation. When we add those foods back to the diet 80 out of 100 of my clients find they are sensitive to gluten.

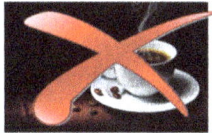

Coffee — Both caffeine and coffee have been shown to lower estrogen levels. A couple of great alternatives include a product called Dandy Blend and another called Teeccino. Dandy Blend is made of water-soluble extracts of roasted roots of dandelion, chicory and beets, and the grains of barley and rye. I also like Teeccino which is a chicory blend herbal tea. Both are gluten free and promote digestive health. Dandy Blend is great support for your liver which is where estrogen gets metabolized and Teeccino is a good source of inulin, a prebiotic soluble fiber, which feeds your gut flora.

Foods that can increase healthy estrogen levels:

Studies conducted by the Linus Pauling Institute of Oregon State University indicated that eating plant-based foods that contain phytoestrogens may help women raise estrogen levels. Phytoestrogens are a group of natural estrogen receptor modulators found in various foods.

Seeds – Flaxseeds and sesame seeds

Fruit – Apricots, oranges, strawberries, peaches, dried prunes, pomegranate

Vegetables – Yams, carrots, alfalfa sprouts, kale, celery

Soy – Old fashioned soy such as miso, tempeh, natto, tofu and soy sauce/tamari (unprocessed or non-GMO soy)

Dark rye bread – Careful, it contains gluten

Legumes – Lentils, peas, pinto beans

Olives and olive oil

Chickpeas

Culinary/Therapeutic herbs – Turmeric, thyme, sage, maca

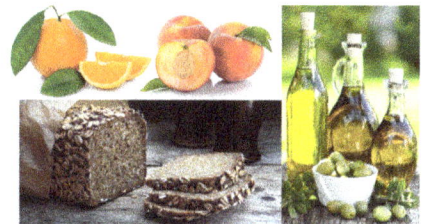

It's simple to incorporate these foods in your daily life. Flaxseeds can be added to smoothies, soups, salads and casseroles. Sesame seeds are a great addition to cooked veggies. You can make a simple salad dressing using miso. Peas and beans are a cinch to add to salads and soups or just eat some hummus as a health snack with cut up veggies. I also love a "mocktail" of grapefruit seltzer, about an ounce of pomegranate juice and fresh squeezed lime with a drop of doTerra lime essential oil. Keep it simple and use your creativity.

A word about Maca

Maca is known as "Peruvian Ginseng" although it is not related to ginseng. But like ginseng it increases strength, energy, and stamina. Studies show that maca can increase libido as well as fertility. It's also helpful for post-menopausal symptoms like insomnia, poor memory, mood issues and hot flashes.

A couple of years ago I had some extensive dental work done. It made me feel like someone had knocked the stuffing out of me. I just couldn't get out of my own way. My energy had deserted me. So, I started to take maca. Within a month I was back to my old self again.

I recommend that you go slow. Start with about ¼ teaspoon per day and increase up to about 1 tablespoon. Some people love it, but others get digestive side effects. Make sure you are using a high quality maca which is gelatinized.

What about soy?

You can't talk about phytoestrogens without having a conversation about soy. I believe soy has been maligned over the past decade. So, let's dive into it with the goal of helping you with any confusion you may have about soy and give you some practical advice on whether and how to eat soy safely.

Are there health benefits to eating soy?

The answer to this is an emphatic yes! Let's talk about breast cancer prevention, first. Asian women who have consumed traditional soy products since childhood or adolescence have significantly lower rates of breast cancer. Some studies have been conflicting, but analysis of large studies say soy consumption either has some positive effect on breast cancer prevention or no effect at all, but it does not pose a risk.

The protective effects of soy are attributed to isoflavones which belong to a class of substances called phytoestrogens. Phytoestrogens are weaker than human estrogen but provide competition at estrogen receptor sites which blocks the effect of the stronger estrogen and keeps them from creating cancerous changes in tissue.

Soy also can be very helpful for menopausal symptoms, particularly hot flashes. Once again this is due to the phytoestrogens.

Several studies have also found that genistein, which is also an isoflavone, may help to reduce bone loss. Finally, there is good reliable research about the cholesterol lowering effect of soy. But to be clear, a plant-based diet will give you the same effects, but soy is an easy addition, in moderation, for variety.

But here is the rub.

You need to know what type of soy and how much. There are several different kinds of soy in our food supply: traditional, processed and GMO soy.

Traditional soy includes foods such as tempeh, natto, miso, and tamari which are also fermented foods. Tofu, edamame and soymilk fall into this category as well. These foods in the US are generally made from non-GMO soy. They are considered real food and a great choice if you would like to add some soy to your diet.

Highly processed soy which is marketed as meat and dairy substitutes such as soy cheese, tofu hot dogs, soy yogurt, soy ice cream, soy bacon, soy sausage links, and soy burgers are not a good choice. Processing of the soy destroys phytonutrients and phytoestrogens. This is the same as eating junk food. Soy protein isolates used in protein powders and protein bars fall into this category.

Increasingly, refined soy foods – things like soy concentrates, textured soy, soy lecithin, etc. – are finding their way into our shopping baskets. It is estimated that between 2000 and 2007, United States food manufacturers introduced over 2,700 new foods with soy as an ingredient. And most of the soy foods being sold in North America are heavily processed. And created from GMO soy.

GMO soy is challenging to avoid. Soybeans are the number one genetically modified food and over 90% of the soy produced in the US food supply is genetically modified. I know some say genetically modified foods are not a problem but I have been in the nutrition field for over 40 years and am seasoned enough to have seen issues like Roundup® scientifically accepted as safe only to find out not too many years later that it causes cancer and profound changes in the gut microbiome.

Stick with the traditional sources of soy outlined above. Also, the best way to be sure your soy products are non GMO is to look for the butterfly on packaging that indicates Non-GMO Project verification. If you want it organic too, look for the USDA Organic label because they are not the same.

How much soy is healthy?

Moderation is the key. Soy should be eaten as a complement to your diet not a mainstay. Two to three servings per week is a good goal.

Some cautions about soy

Breast tumors-- Due to tofu's weak hormonal effects, some doctors tell women with estrogen-sensitive breast tumors to avoid or limit their soy intake. If you are uncomfortable eating soy, don't eat it.

Thyroid issues--Some professionals also advise individuals with poor thyroid function to avoid tofu due to its impact on thyroid function. I agree with this.

Soy is a healthy food for most people to add to their diet for variety. Just make sure you know what you are eating and don't overdo it.

Thyroid Balance

Your thyroid is a small butterfly shaped organ at the base of your throat. It may be small, but the thyroid is one of the most important organs in the body because it regulates every cell. Thyroid fatigue impacts metabolic rate, sex hormone levels, overall mood, wellbeing, and the ability to build muscle.

Many of my clients suffer from underactive thyroid which is grossly underdiagnosed. You may have gone to see your doctor with complaints of fatigue, difficulty losing weight, dry skin, aching joints and digestive issues only to be told that you are just getting older. This is unacceptable! First, who wants to hear that? But more importantly, it's not just aging. Estimates are that over 10% of the population has undiagnosed thyroid problems and it may be as high as 65% in people aged 40 and older.

Some doctors are well intentioned but underinformed. Many believe that an evaluation of thyroid stimulating hormone (TSH) is enough to determine if further testing is needed to evaluate your thyroid. But TSH is just the tip of the iceberg.

TSH levels reflect your pituitary gland communicating to your thyroid that more thyroid hormone is needed. It is not a measure of your actual thyroid hormone levels, how well they are being manufactured, or how well they are being converted to more active levels of thyroid hormone. To figure this out we need to dig deeper and look at your total and free T3 and T4 as well as your thyroid antibodies.

For example, you could have normal TSH levels but a low amount of free T3 which is the active form of thyroid hormone. Or you could have elevated levels of thyroid antibodies which would be indicative of Hashimoto's disease. Hashimoto's is a condition in which your immune system attacks your thyroid leading to inflammation and hypothyroid (underactive thyroid).

I often see clients that have diagnosed hypothyroid but have never had their thyroid antibodies tested to determine Hashimoto's. Hashimoto's is an autoimmune disorder which largely goes undiagnosed. If you have hypothyroid, get your antibodies checked. Ask for Thyroid Peroxidase Antibody (TPO Ab) and Thyroglobulin Antibodies (TgAb). An autoimmune diet protocol is vital to get to the root cause of the disease, inflammation. Although this diet is beyond the scope of this book, I do suggest that you work with a qualified Registered Dietitian Nutritionist or Functional Nutritionist to help you. It could make a major difference in the course of your disease.

The second challenge to getting a good read on your thyroid is that some clinicians are using outdated reference ranges. Most practitioners don't look deeper unless a TSH is greater than 4. I would suggest that you consider 2.5 as the cutoff value.

If you are suffering from any of the symptoms outlined above it would be in your best interest to **know your numbers.** You deserve answers about the cause of your symptoms.

Most of my clients have thyroid challenges ranging from Hashimoto's to hypothyroid to sluggish thyroid. Because the thyroid is dependent on several nutrients to function properly, our work is to deeply nourish the thyroid with a nutrient dense diet.

At the same time, we also look at what is happening with other hormones such as cortisol and estrogen. Remember the adrenals and cortisol are all about survival of the fittest so they get top priority when it comes to resources. As a result, the thyroid doesn't always get what it needs. To heal the thyroid, we need to heal the adrenals. Excess estrogen levels also directly affect the thyroid by hindering its ability to create hormones. Everything is connected when it comes to your hormones. This is one of the reasons why diet as a holistic treatment is so effective. Check out the sections above on how to support the adrenals and reverse estrogen dominance.

Nutrition for your thyroid

Eat a nutrient dense diet focusing on iodine, copper, zinc, selenium and vitamin A.

The **Mindful Menu Plans in Part III** of this book are designed to be nutrient dense in order to support your healing process.

- ❖ Good sources of **Iodine**
  - ➢ Sea vegetables — kombu/kelp, wakame, and arame limited to 1 tsp per day
  - ➢ Saltwater fish and other seafood:
    - ▪ Cod and scallops — excellent
    - ▪ Shrimp — very good
    - ▪ Sardines, salmon, tuna — good sources
  - ➢ Iodized sea salt
- ❖ Good sources of **Copper** — Oysters, mushrooms, seeds, nuts, prunes, dried peas and beans, avocados, goat cheese
- ❖ Good Sources of **Zinc** — Oysters, beef, lamb, wheat germ, spinach, seeds, nuts (particularly cashews), cocoa and chocolate, pork and chicken, grains and legumes
- ❖ Good sources of **Selenium** — Brazil nuts, seafood (particularly oysters), fish, seeds, lean pork, beef, lamb, chicken, turkey, mushrooms
- ❖ Good sources of **Vitamin A** — Sweet potato, carrots, dark leafy greens, squash, romaine lettuce, apricots, cantaloupe, sweet red peppers, mango

Limit some foods

Some healthy foods called goitrogens can interfere with the function of your thyroid. If you have thyroid challenges, it is best to avoid these foods. If your thyroid is healthy, the health benefits of these foods far outweigh any negative effect on your thyroid so go ahead and enjoy them.

- ❖ Raw cruciferous vegetables: Broccoli, kale, spinach, cabbage, etc. — steamed is fine
- ❖ Foods that contain gluten
- ❖ Soy foods: Tofu, tempeh, edamame beans, soymilk, processed soy
- ❖ Certain fruits: Peaches, pears, strawberries

Avoid toxins

Your thyroid is very sensitive to toxins. Everyone is different so there are different tolerances. Do your best to avoid:

- ❖ Unsafe cosmetics
- ❖ Unfiltered water
- ❖ Heavy metals (e.g., mercury in tuna)
- ❖ Bromine, chlorine and fluoride (e.g., bromine is in bleached flour)
- ❖ Cleaning fluids
- ❖ Pesticides and herbicides
- ❖ Non-stick cookware
- ❖ Flame retardants
- ❖ Plastics
- ❖ Xenoestrogens (outlined above)

EC came to see me when she was 60 years old. Her hypothyroid disease had been diagnosed over 30 years ago. She complained of fatigue, autoimmune issues, digestive challenges, insomnia, joint pain and mood issues. She was on multiple medications, suffered from multiple allergies, and had restless leg syndrome.

Her cortisol levels were unbalanced. She was estrogen deficient and her thyroid was sluggish. Within just 3 months after following a diet which addressed her food sensitivities, supported her thyroid and adrenals, adequate water, and gut healing, she had lost about 10 pounds, reduced her need for meds, her insomnia improved, and she felt much more energetic.

Chapter 12
Improve Your Gut Health

It's very simple. Your gut either keeps you healthy or it makes you ill. A healthy gut determines which nutrients to absorb and does an expert job keeping toxins, allergens, and microbes out. An unhealthy gut contributes to a wide range of diseases including diabetes, obesity, rheumatoid arthritis, autism, and depression.

Some 100 trillion organisms reside in your gut, your mouth, and on your skin and are known as your microbiome. This microbiome we carry around with us contains over 500 bacterial species some of which are friendly and others which are not so friendly.

The more we can do to improve the ratio of good bacteria to unhealthy bacteria in our gut the better it is for our overall health. The Human Microbiome Project, a National Institutes of Health initiative, has found that gut imbalances can cause moodiness, low energy, brain fog, gas, joint pain, vitamin and mineral deficiencies, and may even be associated with weight issues.

Here are some factors that cause us to be out of balance:
- Antibiotics and other medications like birth control pills and NSAIDs
- Consumption of conventional farm animal meats due to antibiotic exposure
- Anti-inflammatories (e.g., Aspirin, Ibuprofen, Tylenol, etc.)
- Diets high in refined carbohydrates, sugar, and processed foods
- Diets low in fermentable fibers
- Potential dietary toxins like wheat and dairy
- Chronic stress
- Chronic infections

In fact, just about anyone who lives in the modern world has some level of gut dysfunction. If you never experience stress, please raise your hand!

Did you know that your microbiome is considered an organ? The microbiome is the genetic material of all the microbes - bacteria, fungi, protozoa and viruses - that live on and inside the human body. This microbiome helps us to digest food, protect our immune system and brain, protects us against unhealthy bacteria, and helps to balance hormones. It produces and secretes hormones, regulates the expression of your genes, and exerts control over neurotransmitter and hormones.

And did you know that approximately **80% of your immune system resides in your gut**? Yup. So, if your gut is not healthy it is likely that your immune system isn't either. You may remember that the issue that got me to take my reversal in health so seriously was my bout with Acute Asthmatic Bronchitis twice in one year.

It was particularly puzzling as I had experienced an ironclad immune system for my whole life. Like never more than one cold per decade. My sensitivity to gluten was wreaking havoc with my gut and I just didn't know it. But not being able to breathe got my attention and gave me the inspiration to figure out what was wrong with me.

Having a healthy gut is the #1 key to balancing your hormones because the microbiome is more powerful than all your hormone glands put together.

Here are some good examples of how the gut influences how we look and feel.

Serotonin, the "feel good" neurotransmitter, is produced in the digestive tract. In fact, 90% of all serotonin produced in our body comes from the gut. Serotonin helps to regulate communication between the gut and the brain. It alters our parasympathetic nervous system which can impact our sleep, mood and ability to relax. Serotonin also plays a role in the movement of our gut. So, it can be a factor in such issues as indigestion and constipation.

Another neurotransmitter affected by the gut is dopamine. Dopamine is linked to the reward centers in the brain. When levels of dopamine are low this can have a profound impact on your mood.

In addition, a certain set of your gut bacteria is responsible for metabolizing estrogen. This is called the estrobolome. When your estrobolome is unbalanced, it can lead to excess estrogen which is associated with estrogen dominance and increased risk for breast cancer.

If you have been dealing with brain fog or you feel distracted, it may be challenging to grasp all this information. Just flip ahead to try the Mindful Menus and Recipes in Part III and try the Hormone Balancing Smoothies. You can come back to this at a later time when it will be easier to deal with.

I think it is fair to say that it is practically impossible in the modern world with our exposure to stress, toxins and genetically modified foods, to maintain a healthy gut microbiome. The key is to make sure you have a higher ratio of healthy bacteria (known as probiotics) to unhealthy bacteria such as e. coli and c. diff. And that you have lots of diversity when it comes to your healthy bacteria. This takes some work!

Many of the 10 High Impact Nutritional Strategies to Renew Vitality that are the foundation of this book help to improve healthy bacteria populations in your gut. A powerful step is to avoid refined carbs. I know this is starting to sound like a broken record, but do you get it 100% yet? Unhealthy bacteria love to feed on sugar.

Getting your fiber fix is also smart when it comes to your gut. Fiber feeds the healthy bacteria. But with new research we have learned a lot more about fiber and the different types that feed your gut. One particularly significant type is known as resistant starch. These are foods that are resistant to the digestive process. They are fermented in your colon by your gut bacteria to create short chain fatty acids (SCFA's). SCFA's play an important role in providing an energy source for the cells of the colon. They are also anti-inflammatory, anti-carcinogenic and help us do a better job absorbing minerals while inhibiting the growth of bad bacteria. Check out the table Specific Foods for Your Gut Health below.

You also want to eat more prebiotic and fermented foods. Prebiotics are food for the probiotics (healthy bacteria). Eating more will help to nurture your healthy bacteria. Fermented foods are easy to incorporate into your routine. All you need is about 2 to 4 Tablespoons of fermented food per day. Just be careful what you are buying. Make sure the label says "raw", "fermented" or "brined". The best place to find these foods is in the deli refrigerator. Make sure vinegar is not added to the brine as it destroys the healthy bugs. If you tolerate dairy, yogurt and kefir can be good sources.

Be careful with prepared and processed foods. If you can't pronounce an ingredient in a food your gut won't recognize it either. Also, some additives and preservatives are damaging to your gut. The processing also removes fiber from foods.

Finally, consider taking a probiotic. If you live in the modern world you likely need one. Look for a brand with multiple strains and at least 20 billion colony forming units (CFU's).

SPECIFIC FOODS FOR YOUR GUT HEALTH

Resistant starch
green bananas, green peas, lentils and beans, uncooked rolled oats, and some types of cooked then cooled foods such as potatoes and rice

Prebiotics
oats, onions, leeks, asparagus, Jerusalem artichokes (aka sunchokes) and chicory

Fermented foods
pickles, sauerkraut or any fermented vegetable, kimchi, kombucha, fermented miso, and tempeh

You will find that almost all the recipes in Part III of this book are based on whole foods filled with fiber to assure blood sugar balance, nutrient density, and a healthy gut.

Chapter 13
Limit Stimulants
Caffeine, Alcohol, Stress and Toxins

We have already discussed several powerful things to consider removing including sugar, refined carbs and even dairy and gluten or other substances like soy, corn and eggs if they make you symptomatic.

Other substances that it makes sense to either avoid or start limiting in your life include **caffeine, alcohol, stress and toxins**. Let's start with coffee because this is one of the challenging substances to give up. It can be particularly difficult if you have been suffering fatigue or low energy. In our culture we tend to use coffee or other caffeine substances as drugs to keep us going.

Not everyone needs to quit caffeine

Some of us metabolize caffeine quickly and others are slow metabolizers. You are a slow metabolizer if you find yourself jittery for hours on 1 to 2 cups of coffee. This is likely due to a minor gene mutation which doesn't allow your liver to detox as effectively as others. You might find that a switch to tea helps you to feel calmer and more centered.

Healing Your Adrenals

I think it is fair to say that about 90% of the clients that come to see me for nutrition services have high cortisol levels. Caffeine is a stimulant. This is one of the reasons we depend on it. For many people, every time they drink a cup of coffee or caffeinated soft drink, it causes the flight or fight response which causes increased cortisol. If you are trying to heal your adrenal glands, coffee needs to go.

The best strategy for this is to wean yourself off your cup of Joe. If you go cold turkey, you may feel miserable — vicious headaches, exhausted and maybe even irritable. In fact, you may have tried to quit before and stopped precisely because of these symptoms. Just go slow on this.

Let's say you drink three cups of coffee per day. For your first week or less reduce your consumption to 2 cups per day. Then you can cut back to 1½ cups for a few days when you can drop it to 1 cup per day. Congratulate yourself on some great progress. Just keep going by reducing your intake by ½ every few days. By the time you are drinking a ¼ cup of coffee you will wonder why you are even bothering.

Saying goodbye to coffee is an important step you can take to heal your adrenals. As mentioned in the section of Post-Menopausal Vitality, great substitutes for coffee include Teeccino, Roasted Dandelion Tea and Dandy Blend which taste great and can also make a positive impact on your digestive health.

Estrogen and caffeine

Some other reasons for considering quitting caffeine are estrogen and thyroid. Some preliminary research indicates that caffeine does affect your estrogen level. Both estrogen and caffeine are metabolized by the liver, so they compete with one another for elimination. As a result, you may not be eliminating estrogen properly which can contribute to estrogen dominance. If that is a concern for you, limiting caffeine would be a good choice. If you remember, estrogen dominance can interfere with your thyroid by making hormone receptors less sensitive and blocking the conversion of thyroid hormone to its more active form.

Dehydration and mineral loss

Caffeine is dehydrating. If you feel challenged to get half of your body weight in ounces of water daily, you may consider cutting back on caffeine. It is also nutrient-depleting, particularly vitamins and minerals needed by the hormone challenged body such as B6, magnesium, calcium, iron and other B vitamins.

What about tea?

When it comes to caffeine, the main difference between coffee and tea is the amount. Coffee contains about 200 mg per cup while tea is more like 20 to 60 mg per cup. That is a big difference. Tea also includes L-theanine which can help you feel more alert yet calm at the same time.

Alcohol

Light to moderate alcohol intake can have an anti-inflammatory effect but heavy alcohol use causes intestinal inflammation. Light to moderate means one drink per day for women and up to 2 drinks per day for men. A drink is defined as 12 ounces of beer, 5 ounces of wine and 1.5 ounces of liquor.

Have you noticed how wineglasses have grown larger over the last 20 years? Seriously, when I look at the wineglasses I received for a wedding present 30 years ago, I inevitably reach for the water goblet because it's larger! It is easy to get 3 or even 4 times the recommendation when it comes to alcohol.

Alcohol can be a slippery slope. First, alcohol is empty calories which means you get the fuel without any nutrients. Secondly, alcohol is preferentially metabolized by the liver which means other sources of fuel such as glucose and fat are waiting around to be used and can end up as fat. This usually gets laid down as belly fat. Alcohol can also affect your judgement which may lead to more consumption of inflammatory foods such as sugar or even more alcohol.

In addition, alcohol interferes with a good night sleep. Research indicates increased periods of wakefulness during sleep cycles with alcohol consumption. Since sleeping is one of the most healing things you can do for your inflammation and hormones, it needs to be a priority. Unfortunately, many of us don't get the suggested 7.5 to 9 hours a night. Try looking at your alcohol consumption with a clear eye.

Finally, alcohol interferes with digestion. This can lead to impaired digestion and malabsorption of nutrients. We have talked about the importance of gut health extensively in this book. It's a key to hormone and inflammation balance.

Stick to one drink three times a week or less to keep your inflammation low. Intermittent drinking is better for your long-term health than regular consumption. Give your liver a rest and try a mocktail instead (there are several great mocktail recipes in the Beverages section in Part III).

And when you do choose to have an alcoholic drink, it really matters what you put in the glass. Sugary drinks like Margaritas and some of the fancy martinis offered are off the charts when it comes to sugar. Better choices include a dry wine or vodka, tequila or whiskey on the rocks sipped very slowly or with seltzer.

Think of it this way. Coffee drinking and alcohol are like sacred ceremonies in our lives. Many people feel it is challenging to get the day off to a good start without their morning brew. And most women I know don't feel like they can truly relax in the evening until they have a glass of wine in their hand. It's our favorite cue to put our feet up at the end of the day. But when you think about it, most of us taste the first sip or two and that's it. We aren't paying attention. I recommend that you still take out the beautiful wine glass or favorite mug. Just fill it with something that will be better for your health.

A glass of wine, a cup of coffee — these are things that help us relax and enjoy life. But since both coffee and alcohol tend to cause hormone imbalance, cutting back just makes sense. An occasional cup of coffee or glass of wine is not a problem. The problem occurs when you use these substances to manage your mood or your energy level. Try more productive alternative behaviors like deep breathing, a little stretching, or go for a walk in nature.

Stress

Along with gut challenges, stress is a root cause of hormone imbalance and excess inflammation. Stress has an impact on every single one of the hormone systems that we have reviewed. In addition, when you are stressed it increases oxidative stress in your body leading to inflammation.

When you think about the world we live in with constant noise, light, interruptions from all our devices, constant deadlines, expectations from families and loved ones, we are all stressed. Even those of us who do not feel stressed are living under a certain amount of pressure.

Look at it this way. At least in the US culture, we are constantly at a level of moderate stress — just because we live here. Then add your own personal stress to that burden. Our stress levels are off the charts!!

It is very simple. If you aren't engaged in something you love that helps you manage your stress, it is highly likely that you will not heal your hormones and inflammation.

There are lots of great resources to help you get your stress under better control such as yoga, meditation, prayer, regular massage, deep breathing, consistent exercise, reflexology, reiki and self-hypnosis. Everyone is different. Find something that works for you.

Toxins

Environmental toxins are a major source of inflammation and hormone imbalance. They are everywhere — in the water we drink, the air we breathe, and the food we eat. The more conscious you become the more you can decrease your toxin exposure.

Here are some healthy changes to make if you haven't already:

1. **Avoid heavy metals** — Mercury is high in large predator fish like king mackerel, marlin, orange roughy, shark, swordfish, tilefish, and ahi tuna. Be careful of sushi, too. You can reduce mercury

exposure from sushi by holding back on all types of tuna, mackerel, sea bass, and yellowtail. Other heavy metals include lead, cadmium and arsenic. Filtered water and air are effective ways to reduce heavy metal exposure.

2. **Choose non-toxic cleaning and personal care products** — Did you know that a woman on average applies around 16 personal care products every morning? Many of these substances are toxic and can interfere with hormones as well as cause inflammation. I love the Beautycounter® line because the company has made a major commitment to keeping toxins out of their products.

3. **Eat organic** as much as you can. The Environmental Working Group guidelines are very helpful at: www.ewg.org.

4. **Avoid xenoestrogens** as outline in Chapter 11 – Eat for Hormone Balance. These substances are known estrogen disrupters. They can mimic or partly mimic naturally occurring hormones. They can also bind at the hormone receptor site blocking the body's own estrogen. Or, they can interfere with the way hormones or their receptors are made. To keep it simple, they act somewhat like estrogen, but they don't really do the job.

5. **Get rid of plastic** — Plastic is not good for your health or the environment. It is a source of BPA, another estrogen disrupter. Thyroid hormones are altered by BPA and there is growing evidence that risk of obesity and diabetes is associated with BPA.

These chapters on the 10 High Impact Nutritional Strategies have given you some important advice on what makes up a healthy diet. In the next chapter we will talk about how to deal with cravings. We all get them at least some of the time. It helps to know why they happen and what you can do to control them.

Chapter 14
Manage Cravings

What is a craving?

To crave something means to have a strong desire for it. Sometimes it feels like this desire is totally uncontrollable and will not be satisfied until you get that specific food. But the truth is that cravings generally only last for 5 to 10 minutes at the most.

It's different for everyone but cravings are usually for junk food, sugar, fats and salt. This can be a major obstacle to taking on a healthier eating style.

But here is the good news. Some people think that cravings will build in intensity until they become overwhelming. But cravings are more like waves. They build, crest and then they disappear. Sometimes the best strategy is to relax and wait ten minutes.

Why do we get cravings?

Scientists are still working on piecing together the puzzle around how to conquer cravings. Some of it is related to hormones and some to mindless eating. One thing we know for sure is that every craving starts with a cue.

Any cue that is associated repeatedly with a food can create a craving. For example, you might have been brought up on your mother's homemade chocolate chip cookies which were associated with comfort. As an adult, you will very likely crave chocolate chip cookies when you are stressed and need comfort.

When you satisfy the craving (with cookies or sweets) it activates the brain's pleasure center which releases dopamine. Dopamine is the neurotransmitter that is associated with reward. It creates a rush of euphoria that the brain seeks over and over again. So, it's not about willpower. It's a physiological response.

At the same time, your brain starts to convince you that you are starving. Seems devious, doesn't it? Ghrelin, which is the hunger hormone, increases and insulin decreases both of which make you hungrier. So, when you are presented with a plate of chocolate chip cookies, it becomes impossible to eat just one. You may have noticed that the pact that you make with yourself to just have one itty bitty piece really doesn't work.

And it's not helpful that the dopamine response starts immediately while satiety signals can kick in more slowly. This may seem incredibly maladaptive but back in caveman days it was necessary for survival of the fittest. It helped us to remember to get hunting and gathering for nutrient and calorie dense foods. But here is the rub. In today's environment food is everywhere! People are talking about it, you can smell it or see it in person, on television, on the internet or in a magazine. It's all around. And manufacturers know exactly how much salt, sugar and fat will get your cravings going.

Another theory involves the neurotransmitter, serotonin. Serotonin is also known as the "feel good neurotransmitter" but it, too, is involved in satiety. When serotonin levels are low it can trigger the desire to eat more and create food cravings for foods like refined carbs and sugar.

The challenge is to make sure that your diet facilitates mental wellbeing by keeping your serotonin at healthy levels. You can boost serotonin with healthy carbs like root vegetables and fresh fruit. Some great choices to keep you well-nourished and hopefully away from sugar and refined carbs include beets, carrots, parsnips, rutabaga, sweet potatoes, berries, apples, pears, figs and other fruits. Sunshine helps increase serotonin too!

How to better manage cravings

Eat regularly – Your body needs fuel to keep it going. If you skip meals allowing yourself to get overly hungry, it's difficult to control cravings. Regular balanced meals which contain carbs, protein and fat will keep you satisfied for longer.

Protein – Protein appears to jack up the levels of dopamine in your brain, which helps quell your unhealthy cravings. This is especially true about breakfast. We often find ourselves rushing to get out the door in the morning so many of us neglect a protein-packed breakfast. As a result, we experience midmorning cravings for sugary foods like donuts, pastries or even a bagel.

Following the recommendation of at least 2 to 3 ounces of protein for breakfast, lunch and dinner will be helpful to balance your blood sugar, your energy, and your cravings. For example, if you have a high protein breakfast (e.g., Smoothie or Baked Egg Cups) it will make it easier for you to avoid the pastries at work in the morning. If you do have cravings, you need to check in with yourself. Are you stressed? Do you really feel hungry? Is it just the presence of the pastry that caused the craving? This is mindfulness. Ask yourself what is at the root of your craving.

Healthy Fats – Fats can also help to control cravings. If you are dealing with a craving that just won't quit, try some almond butter smeared on a piece of fruit. It's yummy and will help your craving pass.

Sleep – Research constantly links less sleep and low serotonin levels which leads to cravings for sugary foods. Also, if you have not slept well, before you even start your day your hormones are already unbalanced. You may find yourself craving carbs all day.

Stress – It is well-known that we are hard wired to go for sugar, unhealthy fat and salt when we are stressed. Better stress management is key to craving control.

Hydrate – Hydration is important to conquering your cravings. It can be hard to distinguish between dehydration and hunger. If you aren't conscious of this link, it is easy to mistake thirst for hunger.

Recent research says that 75% of us exist in a state of mild dehydration. Dehydration can also make it difficult for your liver to release glycogen and other forms of stored fuel. The liver depends on water to facilitate these reactions. Dehydration results in a lack of energy and low blood sugar which makes you feel hungry and increases cravings.

Being dehydrated can also interfere with brain levels of serotonin. Try asking yourself, "Am I hungry, or just thirsty?" Drink a glass of water first. If you still feel hungry in 20 minutes, then it makes sense to have something to eat.

Distract yourself – Set your timer and do something to distract yourself. Experts say that most cravings are short lived. Do something you love for 10 minutes and you will be surprised how easy it is to lose your hankering for something unhealthy.

Learn how to nurture yourself – We have learned to associate feel good moments with certain foods of childhood, so we like to turn to them for an emotional pick me up. It's not the food so much as the emotion we tend to associate with it. You don't want the cookies your mom used to bake so much as the love and care associated with every cookie. In fact, what you are looking for is nurturing.

I often ask my clients a question which is often met with complete silence and that is "What nurtures you?" They generally don't have an answer because they have been too busy taking care of everyone else. A good tactic to conquer cravings is to come up with a list of 5 nurturing activities that have no relationship to food. It's different for each person. Some say deep breathing, others feel that spending time in nature makes a huge difference, while still others are nurtured by music and/or reading or even a bubble bath.

Learning how to distract yourself is a good strategy because cravings are short-lived. Focusing on supreme self-care is even smarter. If you don't take great care of yourself, who will?

Practice mindfulness – Mindfulness refers to being aware and in the moment. Unfortunately, most of us have about ten other things on our minds. We are preoccupied about what happened yesterday and worried about what is going to happen tomorrow. And stressed about what might happen next week.

Being aware helps you to focus on the present moment so you can get more enjoyment out of what you are doing instead of being constantly distracted. Tuning in reminds us to gently bring ourselves back to the present moment.

Try observing yourself. Check in by asking yourself questions. Are you hungry? OR is it stress? Boredom? Restlessness? What is the trigger in your environment that is encouraging you to eat? What does hunger feel like to you? What do you need in this moment? Is it really hunger or an emotional craving? How do you know if you are full?

Journaling or keeping a food diary helps to keep this inner dialogue going. Once you get into a groove of healthy eating you won't need to journal every day. You can use it as a tool when you are struggling and need to get your arms around what is going on with cravings.

Start becoming conscious of what drives your behavior. You don't have to be swept away by your impulses. Instead you will see that you have the choice to respond with foresight and wisdom rather than habit and reactivity.

Part III

Notes on Mindful Menus

My practice is based on teaching the basics of a healthy eating plan, customizing it to the individual and helping my clients to practice mindfulness. I don't believe in diets because they are restrictive, don't really teach people what they need to know for the long run, and basically aren't fun. If you practice the 10 High Impact Nutrition Strategies to Renew Vitality and pay attention to how you feel and what might be driving you to eat, you will be more successful. This helps you to learn more about yourself and what is the best program for you.

Along those lines, use the Mindful Menus as a guideline. They are not designed to be inflexible. You don't need to grit your teeth and follow everything in the menu. If you do you will just get bored, rebellious and resentful which is not a great place to be to effect change. Instead let your experience be dynamic and based on your preferences.

For example, you may not like fish or perhaps it is salmon that you don't like. No problem. Just check out the other Main Course recipes and find a replacement that you do like. Fish is a great food for your hormones and inflammation. Maybe you can learn to like it over time but don't force yourself. Remember, food should be enjoyable and healthy. As a side note, I think most people don't like fish because it has not been cooked properly. You might just want to try one of the recipes. Either way, it is all good.

Let yourself be led by your experiences and choices. If you let the suggestions strictly drive you it is easy to get into black and white thinking. This is when your thoughts are ruled by "sticking to" which is perceived as success versus "blowing off" the plan which is seen as failure. Thoughts like this won't help you change. It will only frustrate you.

Using mindfulness, which we talk about in the Cravings chapter, pay attention to what you really need. Are you having cravings? Do you need to revamp the plan a bit? You personally may not do well with carbs for breakfast. On the gluten free oatmeal day, you may feel hungry mid-morning. This just may not be enough protein for you. Learn about yourself by taking note of how you feel. You may need to have a light snack or consider avoiding so much carbohydrate for breakfast.

Following your plan can free up mental energy and reduce stress around food. With a plan you can feel more empowered and able to make better decisions about what you need to nourish your body.

Portion Control

You may have noticed that I have not included portion sizes in the menus. First, I don't know what you need daily to keep you fueled because we are all different. But more importantly, this feels more like a "diet" than a moving toward a healthy eating style. As I mentioned before, it is a good practice to strive for about 2 to 3 ounces of protein per meal. If you are trying to lose weight, it makes sense to cut back on carbs like sweet potato, quinoa and brown rice bearing in mind that a serving is about a half cup.

It is far more important to pay attention to your level of hunger. This takes learning the difference between hunger and cravings. Hunger is an actual physiological feeling. Your stomach is rumbling, or you feel lightheaded. Craving, on the other hand, is a strong desire and more psychological.

If you have struggled with your weight, you may not know what hunger really feels like. We often push those feelings away because we don't want to feel hungry. Hunger is a cue to eat which can feel challenging because in the past we have made unhealthy choices.

But hunger can be your friend. It's a mechanism that your body uses to tell you that it is time to eat. The more you can tune in to this and make some healthy choices, the better success you will have.

Meal prep and leftovers

Make this easy on yourself. If you are taking time to create a great dinner for yourself, make plenty so you can either eat or repurpose leftovers. For example, in the Week 2 Menu, you could cook yourself extra scallops on Monday so you can have them on your Spinach Salad for lunch on Tuesday.

It also helps if you do some pre-prep on your veggies when you have some down time. If you know what your meals are going to be you can chop up some onions and other veggies as well as cook a whole grain ahead of time so you can avoid the stressful mad dash to get dinner on the table in the evening during the week. You can store these foods in glass containers with a vacuum top. They will stay fresh for days in your fridge.

You don't need to make a big deal out of dinner every night. Remember the Mindful Menus are there to give you ideas and lots of variety. Burgers made from free range turkey or grass-fed beef nicely seasoned are simple and easy. So is Smoked Paprika Baked Chicken. Just cover half of your plate with a seasonal veggie you love and add some mashed cauliflower seasoned with garlic powder and rosemary or a small serving of grain like quinoa. Dinner is done and you can get on to the next thing.

Keep your kitchen well stocked

Organize your kitchen so you have some shelf-stable choices that you can use in a pinch. I like to keep a couple of different sizes of shrimp in my freezer along with some basic frozen veggies and fruit.

In my pantry, I keep a wide variety of grains, wild rice, dried legumes, nuts, seeds, dried fruit, and gluten free flours. Canned goods include canned tomatoes, tomato paste, reduced-sodium chicken broth, beef broth and/or vegetable broth, clam juice, canned coconut milk for Asian curries, soups and lattes, canned beans like cannellini, chickpeas, black beans, other beans. And cans of chunk light tuna, salmon and sardines are always available for last minute meals

For flavor, I recommend a well-supplied herb and spice cabinet. I always have fresh onions, shallots and garlic on hand along with fresh lemons and limes. Mustard, anchovies, fish sauce, tamari and nut oils reside in my refrigerator. Maple syrup, stevia, cacao nibs and powder as well as dark chocolate are always on hand.

This way I can stay on top of what I have used up during the week and replenish it when I go to the grocery store. It keeps shopping easy because I stick to the periphery where I can find the fresh seasonal food such as fruit, veggies, protein and plant-based milks, such as almond or coconut.

Enjoy your food

Most important is to make your eating experience enjoyable. You can have delicious fabulous meals that are targeted toward balancing hormones and inflammation. Just use the Mindful Menus for direction sprinkled with a healthy dose of your own creativity and ingenuity. Have fun and don't judge yourself harshly. Maybe you try something, and it doesn't turn out perfectly. Just learn what you can from it and move on.

28 DAYS OF MINDFUL MENUS
MINDFUL MENU – WEEK 1

	Breakfast	Lunch	Snack	Dinner
Monday	GF Oatmeal with almond milk, chopped pear and walnuts	Garden Salad with Salmon & black beans, Simple Easy Salad Dressing	Hummus and carrots, celery	Smoky Paprika Baked Chicken Breast, Roasted Root Veggies
Tuesday	Berry Smoothie (customized to hormone need)	Smoked Paprika Baked Chicken Breast (Monday Leftovers)	Turkey Roll-up	Pork Tenderloin with Roasted Apples & Onions, Brown Rice, Roasted Cauliflower
Wednesday	Chia Seed Pudding	Chicken Salad with Avocado Dressing sandwich, Open-faced on GF bread	Turmeric Pumpkin Latte	Pan-Seared Flounder and Green Beans, Cauliflower Mash
Thursday	Cherry Zinger Smoothie	Black Bean Soup	Berries with handful of pecans	Roasted Veggies and Chicken Sausage, Sautéed spinach with garlic
Friday	2 eggs, soft boiled, Avocado slices	Black Bean & Quinoa Salad, grapefruit segments or 2 small tangerines	Trail Mix	Spicy Coconut Salmon, Brown Rice, Broccoli
Saturday	Spicy Coconut Salmon (Friday leftovers)	White Bean & Avocado Salad, Dijon Salad Dressing	Veggies and Red Pepper "Cheese" Dip	Sweet Potato Chili, Garden Salad
Sunday	2 eggs scrambled with onions and mushrooms, slice of GF bread smeared with avocado	Black Bean Soup (Thursday leftovers), Small orange	Tomatoes & Avocado drizzled with olive oil	Roast Cod with Cherry Tomatoes, Olives & Capers Swiss Chard, Quinoa

Snacks only when needed. Pay attention to your level of hunger.

MINDFUL MENU – WEEK 2

	Breakfast	Lunch	Snack	Dinner
Monday	Chai Banana Smoothie	Smart Lentil Soup	Small Handful of Cashews	Pan Seared Scallops with Garlic & Paprika, Miso Glazed Carrots, Tasty Cauliflower Rice
Tuesday	Breakfast Egg Cups	Spinach Salad with leftover Scallops, Dijon Salad Dressing	Hummus with Celery and Jicama	Mushroom Steaks w/ kale and red onion, Sweet Potato, Garden Salad with Good Seasons Italian knockoff dressing
Wednesday	Southern Style Shake	Mushroom Steaks on White Bean & Avocado Salad (Tuesday Leftovers)	Grain Free Granola Bars	Pork tenderloin with Italian herb rub, Roasted Brussels sprouts with Balsamic vinegar, Cauliflower Mash
Thursday	Tofu Scramble, slice of GF bread smeared with avocado	Creamy Cauliflower Soup, fresh pear	Serenity Balls (2)	Turkey Cutlets with Mushrooms & Marsala, Sautéed spinach with garlic, Wild rice
Friday	Southern Style Smoothie	Open Faced Turkey, Tomato & Avocado Sandwich on GF bread (Thursday Leftovers)	Handful of Pecans and Raspberries	Spiced Salmon with Mustard Sauce, Miso Glazed Carrots, Quinoa
Saturday	GF Pumpkin Muffin	Healthy Cobb Salad	Trail Mix	Veggie Curry, Romaine Salad
Sunday	Quinoa Breakfast Skillet	Creamy Cauliflower Soup (Thursday Leftovers), Avocado Prosciutto Roll-up	Handful of Pecans	Chicken in a Pot, GF Fettuccine, Sautéed Kale with garlic

Snacks only when needed. Pay attention to your level of hunger.

MINDFUL MENU – WEEK 3

	Breakfast	Lunch	Snack	Dinner
Monday	Chia Seed Breakfast Pudding	Leftover chicken from Sunday Dinner, Spinach Salad, Sesame Miso Vinaigrette	Golden Milk	Open face Turkey Burger an GF bread, Sliced Tomatoes & avocado
Tuesday	Sunnyside Veggie Eggs with Avocado	Asparagus Quinoa Salad	Black Bean Soup (1 cup portion)	Tandoori Chicken, Quinoa, Sautéed Beet Greens
Wednesday	Banana Ginger Smoothie	Healthy Cobb Salad	Avocado Chocolate Pudding	Broccoli & Zucchini Frittata, GF Roll, Garden Salad, Dijon Salad Dressing
Thursday	Veggie Omelet, Fresh Fruit	Tandoori Chicken (Tuesday Leftovers), green salad	Tofu Snack	Mushroom-Asparagus Risotto, Roasted green beans with garlic, Orange, Beet & Walnut Salad
Friday	Strawberry Kiwi Smoothie	Stir fried Veggies with Tofu	Hummus and cukes	Beef with Bok Choy and Mushrooms, Sweet Potato
Saturday	Tofu Scramble, avocado slices	White Bean & Avocado salad, Champagne Vinaigrette	Stress-Buster Latte	Tenderloin pork with Chicken Sausage and Black Bean Stew, Salad, Dijon Salad Dressing
Sunday	Almond Pancakes, Berries	White Bean, Chicken Sausage & Kale Soup	Guacamole & jicama	Chicken Shish Kabob, Brown Rice, Brussels Sprouts

Snacks only when needed. Pay attention to your level of hunger.

MINDFUL MENU – WEEK 4

	Breakfast	Lunch	Snack	Dinner
Monday	Chicken Shish Kabob, Brown Rice, Brussels Sprouts (Sunday Leftovers)	White Bean, Chicken Sausage & Kale Soup (Sunday Leftovers)	Avocado Prosciutto Roll-Up	Buffalo Burger on Portabella Mushroom, Green Salad, Brown Rice
Tuesday	2 eggs scrambled with onions & mushrooms	Chicken Salad with Avocado Dressing on 1 slice GF bread with tomatoes	Apple with almond butter	Roasted Squash and Mushroom Soup with Chicken Sausage, Tossed Salad, Good Seasons® Italian Dressing Knockoff
Wednesday	GF Oatmeal with berries & pecans, Almond butter	Roasted Squash & Mushroom Soup (Tuesday Leftovers)	Grain Free Granola Bars	Salmon with Miso & Asparagus, Sautéed Spinach with garlic
Thursday	Chai Banana Smoothie	Salmon & Asparagus Salad (Wednesday Leftovers)	Trail Mix	Chickpea Masala, Green Salad, Avocado Dressing
Friday	Hot Quinoa Breakfast cereal with Fruit	Healthy Cobb Salad	Hummus with Endive Scoops	Marinated Shrimp Kabobs, Tasty Cauliflower Rice, Greens with garlic & ginger
Saturday	Pumpkin/Squash Muffin	Shrimp (Friday Leftovers) served on Wilted Asian Salad	Handful of Almonds + Serenity Balls (2)	Spinach & Chickpea Curry, Cauliflower Rice, Roasted Veggies
Sunday	Veggie Omelet, Uncured bacon	Black Bean and Quinoa Salad, Fresh Fruit	Walnuts & Berries	Arugula Salad with Fennel & Roast Salmon

Snacks only when needed. Pay attention to your level of hunger.

RECIPE LIST

APPETIZERS
Spicy Chipotle White Bean Dip
Red Pepper "Cheese" Dip
Roasted Fennel & White Bean Dip
Mushroom Pâté
Baba Ghanoush
Guacamole
Hummus
Shrimp and Guac Bites

BEVERAGES
Golden Milk
Ginger & Turmeric Tea
Hibiscus Tea
Roasted Dandelion Root Latte
Stress-Buster Latte
Turmeric Pumpkin Latte
Alkaline Broth
Pomegranate Lime Spritzer
Coconut, Cucumber, Lime and Mint Cooler
Citrus Basil Seltzer

SALADS
Black Bean and Quinoa Salad
Carrot Salad with Balsamic Vinegar
Brussels Sprouts, Kale and Dried Cranberry Salad
Farro Salad with Peas and Asparagus
Black Bean and Avocado Salad
Asparagus Quinoa Salad
Chicken Salad with Avocado Dressing
Fennel, Orange, Walnut and Arugula Salad
Pomegranate, Beet and Arugula Salad
No-Mayo Coleslaw
Citrus and Broccoli Slaw
Orange, Beet and Walnut Salad
Wilted Asian Salad
Mediterranean Carrot & Chickpea Salad
White Bean and Avocado Salad
Healthy Cobb Salad

SOUPS
Bone Broth
Smart Lentil Soup
Red Bean, Rice and Shrimp Soup
Chicken Vegetable Soup
White Bean, Chicken Sausage and Kale Soup
Creamy Cauliflower Soup
Black Bean Soup
Roasted Squash and Mushroom Soup with Chicken Sausage

Healing Mushroom Soup
Avocado Lime Soup

SIDES
Roasted Brussels Sprouts with Balsamic Vinegar
Roasted Fennel
Roasted Root Veggies
Roasted Summer Veggies
Spicy Cauliflower Pilaf
Cauliflower Mash
Roasted Asparagus with Orange and Walnut
Miso Glazed Carrots
Greens with Garlic and Ginger
Cauliflower with Indian Spices and Pistachios
Roasted Sweet Potatoes, Squash and Arugula
Tasty Cauliflower Rice
Roasted Garlicky Green Beans
Fermented Ginger-Shredded Carrots
Fermented Carrots

SAUCES & DRESSINGS
Sausage Seasoning Blend
Chimichurri Sauce
Veggie Sauce with Miso
Avocado Dressing
Dairy Free Pesto
Cashew Dip
Sesame Miso Vinaigrette
Champagne Vinaigrette Dressing
Dijon Salad Dressing
Tomatillo Salsa
Tahini
Simple Easy Salad Dressing
Good Seasons® Italian Dressing Knockoff
Super Seed Topping

SNACKS
Serenity Balls
Gorp (aka Trail Mix)
Grain-Free Granola Bars
Turkey Roll-Ups
Avocado Prosciutto Roll-Ups
Almond Butter Balls
Roasted Nuts with Herbs
Tofu Snacks

ENTREES
Smoky Paprika Baked Chicken Breast
Tandoori Chicken
Sautéed Chicken with Olives, Capers and Lemons

Roasted Veggies and Chicken Sausage
Grilled Chicken with Garlic Pesto
Turkey Cutlets with Mushrooms & Marsala
Chickpea Masala
Eggplant, Tomato & Chickpea Stew (Slow-Cooker)
Vegetable Curry
Spinach and Chickpea Curry
Shrimp Curry
Buffalo Burger on a Portabella Mushroom
Roast Cod with Cherry Tomatoes, Olives and Capers
Spicy Coconut Salmon with Bok Choy
Arugula Salad with Fennel and Roasted Salmon
Spiced Salmon with Mustard Sauce
Salmon with Crispy Cabbage and Kale
Sesame Encrusted Salmon
Herb-Baked Salmon
Grilled Salmon with Mango Salsa
Shepherd's Pie
Shrimp and Eggplant
Stuffed Sweet Potatoes
Quick Cassoulet
Salmon with Miso and Asparagus
Crispy Baked Tofu
Stir Fried Veggies with Tofu
Chocolate Chili
Beef with Bok Choy and Mushrooms
Shish Kabobs – Chicken/Beef
Pan-Seared Scallops with Garlic and Paprika
Baked Flounder
Pan-Seared Flounder and Green Beans
Codfish with Capers, Lemon and Thyme
Baked Cod with Avocado Salsa
Marinated Shrimp Kebabs
Mushroom Steaks with Kale and Red Onion
Sweet Potato Chili
Chicken in a Pot
Pork Tenderloin with Chicken Sausage and Black Beans
Roasted Pork Tenderloin with Fennel and Garlic
Pork Tenderloin with Roasted Apples and Onions
Pork Tenderloin with Italian Herb Seasoned Rub
Quick Peanut Quinoa Casserole

BREAKFASTS
Autumn Breakfast Casserole
Tofu Scramble
Spring Vegetable Egg Casserole
Broccoli and Zucchini Frittata
Sunnyside Veggie Eggs with Avocado

Kale, Red Onion and Mushroom Frittata
Hormone Balancing Smoothies
Smoothie Recipes
     Detox Berry Smoothie
     Cherry Zinger Smoothie
     Strawberry "Chocolate" Smoothie
     Southern Style Smoothie
     Peach Ginger Smoothie
     Spiced Pumpkin Smoothie
     Banana Ginger Smoothie
     Strawberry Kiwi Smoothie
     Chocolate Cherry Smoothie
     Pina Colada Smoothie
     Chai Banana Smoothie
     Creamsicle Smoothie
Quinoa Breakfast Skillet
Almond Pancakes
Chia Seed Breakfast Pudding
Gluten-Free Pumpkin Muffins
Avocado Toast
Breakfast Egg Cups (To Go)
Healthy Homemade Granola
Hot Quinoa Breakfast Cereal with Fruit
Veggie Omelet

DESSERTS
Coconut "Cookies"
Chocolate Dipped Banana Bites
Dark Chocolate Coconut Bites
Chocolate Avocado Pudding
Cranberry-Apple Crisp
Blueberry and Raspberry Crisp
Healthy Ginger Pumpkin Mousse
Wild Orange Dark Chocolate Dipped Strawberries
Chocolate Cherry Bars

SELECT DAIRY RECIPES
Farro Salad with Peas, Asparagus and Feta
Polenta Bake with Shrimp
Asparagus Quinoa Salad
Eggplant Bundles
Grilled Peaches with Marscarpone Cheese
Chickpea Crust Pizza
Light Chicken Verde Nachos
Smoked Trout Mousse
Spring Vegetable Egg Casserole with Cheese

APPETIZERS

Appetizers aren't always necessary because let's face it many of us are trying to eat less. But if you are entertaining, appetizers are a great way to start off a meal. They don't have to be elaborate. Just having something light to munch on is perfect.

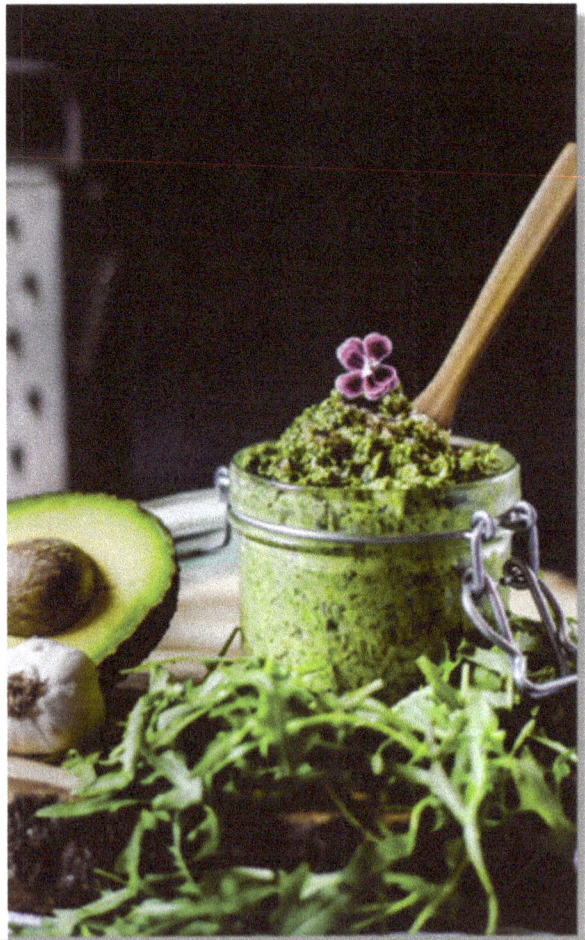

Spicy Chipotle White Bean Dip

I love white beans. They are so adaptable as they soak up the flavors of everything you mix them with. Chipotle adds a smoky flavor which is enhanced by the smoked paprika. Smoked paprika is another favorite spice.

1 15-ounce can cannellini beans, drained
   and rinsed
1-3 chipotle peppers in adobo sauce, or
   more, to taste
2 cloves garlic

2 tablespoons lemon juice
1 teaspoon cumin
1 teaspoon smoked paprika
1 teaspoon chili powder
1/4 cup plus 2 tablespoon olive oil

1. In the bowl of a food processor, combine cannellini beans, chipotle peppers, garlic, lemon juice, cumin, smoked paprika and chili powder.

2. With the motor running, add olive oil in a slow stream until emulsified.

3. Serve with cut-up veggies such as endive or jicama to add variety.

Red Pepper "Cheese" Dip

I am always looking for ways to increase veggies in our diet. This is a delicious creamy dairy free dip that people love. I once took this to a party with a huge platter of veggies and my friends giggled about how large the platter was. Every little bit was gone by the end of the evening.

2 red bell peppers, cut and seeded
1/4 cup fresh lemon juice
3/4 cup nutritional yeast flakes
3/4 cup raw tahini

2 cloves garlic
1½ teaspoons sea salt
1/2 cup water

Servings: makes about 3 cups

1. Throw all the ingredients into a high-speed blender and blend until smooth and creamy.

2. Adjust seasonings to taste, then transfer to bowl and store in the fridge until ready to serve. The cheese sauce will thicken up when chilled, so I recommend chilling the sauce at least an hour or two before serving.

3. Serve with your favorite raw veggies, or chips, and enjoy!

Roasted Fennel & White Bean Dip

Roasted fennel makes this dish special. The flavor is subtle and delish. I suggest that you double the part of the recipe that roasts the fennel and use this for a vegetable in another meal during the week.

1 large or 2 small fennel bulbs, trimmed and cut into 1-inch pieces
2 to 3 tablespoons olive oil
2 cloves garlic, in papery skin
1/2 cup plus 2 tablespoons olive oil
2 garlic cloves, minced

1 15-ounce can of cannellini beans, drained and rinsed
1 tablespoon fresh rosemary, chopped
1 tablespoon lemon juice, fresh
1 teaspoon lemon zest
Carrots sliced lengthwise, endive, zucchini

1. Preheat the oven to 400° F.
2. Toss the fennel and garlic cloves in the 2 tablespoons of olive oil and spread on a sheet pan. Season generously with salt and pepper.
3. Roast for 30-40 minutes, turning twice that time. Take out and let cool.
4. When cool squeeze the roasted garlic out of their skins.
5. In a food processor combine the beans, fresh garlic, rosemary, fennel, roasted garlic, lemon juice and zest, then add remaining ½ cup olive oil. Puree until smooth. Raise oven temp to 450° F. Transfer puree into a small baking dish. Place it on a baking sheet to capture any bubbling over in the oven.
6. Bake about 15 minutes.
7. Serve with cut-up vegetables.

Mushroom Pâté

I love this recipe because it is elegant and great to share when you have company. Mushrooms contain over a dozen vitamins and minerals some of which are powerful antioxidants. They have great umami, one of the five basic tastes, which is best described as savory.

1 teaspoon extra-virgin olive oil plus 2 tablespoons, divided*
1/4 cup minced shallots
1 pound cremini mushrooms (Baby Bella), coarsely chopped
2 tablespoons chopped fresh sage, plus more for garnish

3/4 teaspoon salt
1/4 teaspoon ground pepper
3 tablespoons port or sherry
1/2 cup walnuts, toasted
3 tablespoons nutritional yeast

1. Heat 1 teaspoon oil in a large skillet over medium-high heat.

2. Add shallots and cook, stirring, until starting to lightly brown, about 30 seconds.

3. Add mushrooms and cook, stirring frequently, until their liquid is almost evaporated, 4 to 5 minutes.

4. Add sage, salt and pepper and cook, stirring, for 2 minutes more.

5. Add port or sherry, scraping up any browned bits, and cook until the liquid evaporates, 2 to 3 minutes.

6. Transfer the mixture to a food processor. Add the remaining 2 tablespoons oil, walnuts and nutritional yeast (or Parmesan) and pulse until very finely chopped, about 30 seconds.

7. Serve garnished with sage, if desired.

*You may use clarified butter instead if you wish

Baba Ghanoush

A roasted eggplant dip from Mediterranean cuisine, this dip is easy to make and full of healthy fat from the olive oil and tahini. Tahini is made from ground sesame seeds, so this is a good pick for phytoestrogens which help with low estrogen levels. Plus, cumin is one of my favorite spices. It's easy to use and a little bit packs a lot of flavor.

2 small-to-medium eggplants
2 medium cloves of garlic, pressed or
   minced
2 tablespoons lemon juice, more if
   necessary
1/4 cup tahini

1/3 cup extra-virgin olive oil, plus more
   for brushing the eggplant and
   garnish
2 tablespoons chopped fresh flat-leaf
   parsley, plus extra for garnish
3/4 teaspoon salt, to taste
1/4 teaspoon ground cumin
Pinch of smoked paprika, for garnish

1. Preheat the oven to 425° F with a rack in the upper third of the oven. Line a large, rimmed baking sheet with parchment paper to prevent the eggplant from sticking to the pan.

2. Halve the eggplants lengthwise and brush the cut sides lightly with olive oil. Place them in the prepared pan with the halved sides down.

3. Roast the eggplant, about 35 to 40 minutes. Set the eggplant aside to cool for a few minutes. When cool, scoop out the flesh with a large spoon and discard the skin.

4. Remove as much moisture from the eggplant as you can by placing in a mesh strainer over a mixing bowl. Let the eggplant rest for a few minutes and shake/stir the eggplant to release some more moisture.

5. Drain and wipe out the bowl and place the eggplant into the bowl. Add the garlic and lemon juice to the eggplant and stir vigorously with a fork until eggplant breaks down. Add the tahini and stir. While stirring, slowly drizzle in the olive oil. Continue stirring until the mixture is pale and creamy and use your fork to break up any particularly long strings of eggplant.

6. Stir in the parsley and cumin. Season to taste with more salt and more lemon juice, if desired.

7. Transfer the baba ghanoush to a serving bowl and lightly drizzle olive oil on top. Lastly, sprinkle parsley and smoked paprika on top. Let the baba ghanoush rest for at least 2 hours before serving.

Guacamole

Who doesn't love Guacamole? It, too, is a great party appetizer —delicious and loaded with healthy fats. I like this recipe because it calls for tomatillos which add even more nutrition and flavor to the mix. And I love cilantro! Not everyone does so just use parsley instead if you need to.

3 tomatillos
1/3 cup chopped onion
1/3 cup plum or cherry tomatoes,
    separated from seeds
1/4 cup or more chopped fresh cilantro
2 small jalapeño peppers equivalent
    (from jar), finely chopped

1 tablespoon fresh lime juice
1/2 teaspoon salt
2 ripe* peeled avocados, seeded and
    coarsely mashed
1-2 garlic cloves, minced

1. Peel papery husk from tomatillos; wash, core and finely chop.
2. Coarsely chop the tomatoes.
3. Combine tomatillos, tomatoes, onion and remaining ingredients; stir well.

*If avocados are not ripe when purchased, you can speed up the ripening process by putting them in a sealed brown bag for a day or two.

Hummus

You might be thinking "ho-hum I can get this at the grocery store." Well you can but it won't taste this fresh or good. And it is simple to make with a food processor. The smoked paprika brings the dip up a notch. You can also add additional veggies such as red pepper or artichoke or olives to add more flavor.

1 15-ounce can of chickpeas, drained
1 tablespoon of the liquid reserved
1-2 small garlic cloves, smashed
1 tablespoon fresh lemon juice
1/4 cup tahini sauce

2 tablespoons extra-virgin olive oil
1 teaspoon sweet smoked paprika
Kosher salt
Non-wheat crackers or crudités, for
    serving

1. In a food processor, combine the chickpeas with the liquid, garlic, lemon juice and tahini and puree to a chunky paste.
2. Scrape down the side of the bowl.
3. Add 2 tablespoons of olive oil and the paprika and puree until smooth.
4. Season the hummus with salt, drizzle with olive oil and serve with non-wheat chips/crackers or crudités.

Shrimp and Guac Bites

These are delicious, elegant enough for company or a holiday meal and easy to make.

For Shrimp:

1 lb. medium shrimp, peeled, deveined
  with tail shell removed
1/4 cup extra-virgin olive oil, plus more
  for sautéing shrimp
1/4 cup lime juice (approx. 3 limes)
1 tablespoon brown sugar (or honey)
3 cloves garlic, minced

1 teaspoon smoked paprika, plus more
  for garnish
2 tablespoons hot sauce
(or 1 teaspoon Cajun seasoning & 1/4
  teaspoon cayenne pepper)
Kosher salt

For Guacamole:

1/3 cup finely chopped red onion
1/3 cup plum tomato or cherry tomatoes,
  separated from seeds
1/4 cup or more finely chopped fresh
  cilantro

2 small jalapeño peppers equivalent
  (from jar), finely chopped
1 tablespoon fresh lime juice
1/2 teaspoon salt
2 ripe* peeled & seeded avocados
1-2 garlic cloves, minced

2 medium size cucumbers (may also mix or replace with red pepper)

Servings: 6-8

1. Marinate shrimp: In a medium-size bowl combine olive oil, lime juice, and other ingredients and season with salt to taste. Whisk until fully blended.

2. Add shrimp to marinade and toss until shrimp are thoroughly coated. Cover and refrigerate for 30 min. and no longer than 1 hour (or they will get tough).

3. Make Guac: Coarsely chop the tomatoes. In medium-size bowl mash the avocados with onion, cilantro and other ingredients. Add tomatoes and mix until blended.

4. Prep cucumbers: Peel cucumbers to create striped skin/peel effect. Then slice into ¼"-1/2" rounds. If using red peppers cut into squares approx. 1"-1½".

5. Sauté shrimp in large skillet on medium heat, approx. 2 min. on each side. Remove from heat and allow to cool,

6. On each slice of cucumber (or red pepper) place about 1 tablespoon of guac and then top with a shrimp. Garnish with finely chopped cilantro and/or sprinkled paprika.

*If avocados are not ripe when purchased, you can speed up the ripening process by putting them in a sealed brown bag for a day or two.

BEVERAGES

Beverages not only provide hydration, but they can also be a great source of nutrients. You can add herbs and spices for their balancing effect on hormones and inflammation. Beverages are also a social gathering tool. Share one of these yummy drinks with a friend.

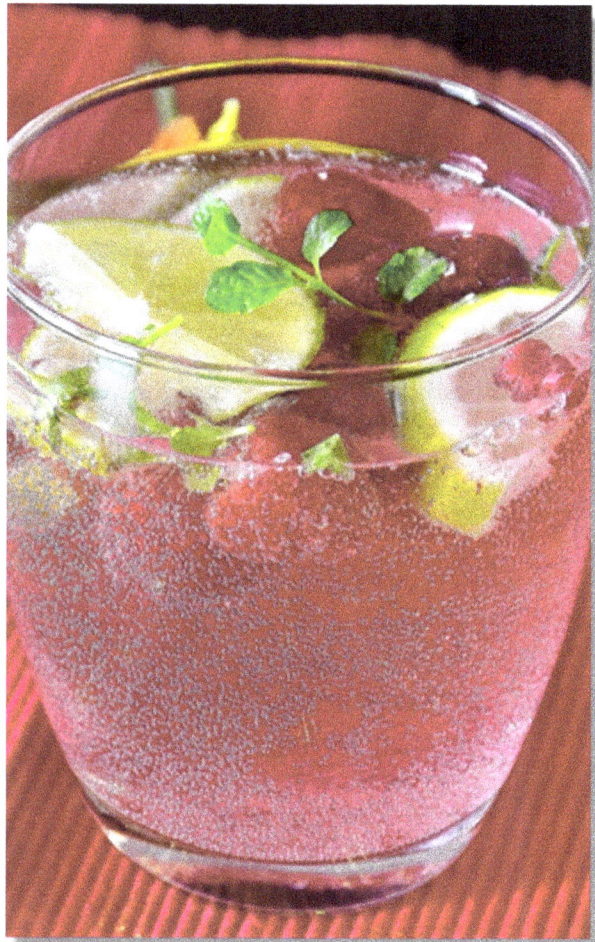

Golden Milk

With turmeric as its main ingredient, this is a highly anti-inflammatory drink. But the best part is that it is warm, spicy and comforting. So great for a cold winter's day.

For the Spice Mix
1/4 cup dried turmeric
1/2 teaspoon black pepper
1 teaspoon cinnamon
1 teaspoon dried ground ginger
1/2 teaspoon ground cardamom
Mix spices together. Store in an airtight container.

For the Golden Milk
1½ cups unsweetened coconut milk
1½ cups almond milk
1 tablespoon spice mix (recipe above)
1 teaspoon coconut oil, olive oil, or ghee
Sweetener of choice (honey, maple syrup, stevia)

1. In a small saucepan, add coconut milk, almond milk, 1 tablespoon Spice Mix, coconut oil, black pepper, and sweetener of choice (I usually add 1 tablespoon (15 ml) maple syrup).

2. Whisk to combine and warm over medium heat. Heat until hot to the touch but not boiling - about 4 minutes - whisking frequently.

3. Turn off heat and taste to adjust flavor. Add more sweetener to taste or more turmeric or ginger for spice.

4. Serve immediately.

Ginger & Turmeric Tea

This tea gives you an anti-inflammatory double whammy with both ginger and turmeric.

1 cup nut or soymilk
1/4 teaspoon ground turmeric
1/4 teaspoon ground ginger
Stevia or monk fruit to taste

1. In a small saucepan, bring milk to a boil.
2. Add turmeric and ginger, reduce heat and simmer for 10 minutes.
3. Strain tea into a cup.
4. Add sweetener and enjoy!

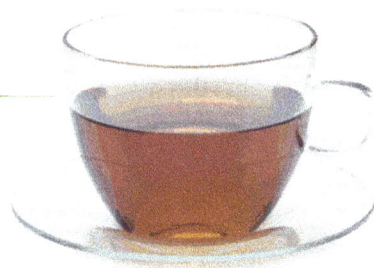

Hibiscus Tea

A tea that is easy to make and a refreshing beverage in the summertime. Great for high blood pressure, too.

1/2 cup dried Hibiscus flowers
8 cups Water
stevia in a dropper

1. Fill a tea kettle with cold water. Once it boils, pour over the Hibiscus flowers.
2. Let it steep for 15 to 20 minutes. Strain the tea. Add stevia for sweetness.
3. You can either serve it warm or refrigerate and serve over ice.

Roasted Dandelion Root Latte

For those of you who want to give your liver some love, this is a great latte. You can also purchase Dandy Blend which is an instant version, and some say tastes like a full-bodied cup of coffee. Either one is a good coffee substitute.

1 cup plant milk such as almond, rice or coconut milk (if you use full fat coconut milk, dilute with 50% water)

1 teaspoon grass fed butter or coconut oil (skip this if you use full fat coconut milk)

1 teaspoon roasted dandelion root powder

1/2 teaspoon cinnamon

1/4 teaspoon cardamom

1/2 teaspoon maple syrup or local honey, raw

1 drop of doTerra Ginger essential oil (optional)

1. Heat the milk in a saucepan on the stove. Add butter or coconut oil if using.

2. Once the added fat is melted, add the dandelion root powder, cinnamon, cardamom and maple syrup, and stir until smooth.

3. Take the mixture off the burner and add the ginger oil.

Stress-Buster Latte

Another calming drink, this elixir is good for your adrenals with the added adaptogens ashwagandha and maca, also known as Peruvian ginseng. Check out my blog at www.smartnutritionblog.com.

1 cup of plant milk, unsweetened—almond, cashew, coconut

1 tablespoon grass fed butter or coconut oil

1 teaspoon ashwagandha root powder*

1/4 teaspoon Maca powder, gelatinized**

1/2 teaspoon Ceylon cinnamon

1/4 teaspoon cardamom

1/2 teaspoon maple syrup or raw honey

1. Warm the milk in a small saucepan on top of the stove. Add the healthy fat.

2. Pour saucepan contents into the blender. Add the powders and maple syrup/honey. Be careful to place the top on the blender loosely and cover with a cloth dish towel—otherwise you will have hot liquid all over you and your kitchen.

3. An alternative to the blender is to use a wire whip and blend all ingredients into the milk mixture.

4. Sit in a comfortable chair. Relax and Enjoy!

* A great source for the ashwagandha and other quality bulk herbs is www.mountainroseherbs.com
** Gelatinized Maca is easier to absorb and you can get it here: www.supplements.smartnutritionllc.com

Turmeric Pumpkin Latte

Chock full of anti-inflammatory spices and delicious too. Great for a cool autumn afternoon snack.

1 teaspoon coconut oil
2 to 3 tablespoons pumpkin purée
1/2 teaspoon ground cinnamon
1/2 teaspoon ground ginger
1/4 teaspoon ground nutmeg

Small pinch of ground allspice
1 teaspoon ground turmeric
1 teaspoon vanilla extract
1 to 2 teaspoons raw local honey
1½ cups reduced fat coconut milk

Servings: 2

1. In a small saucepan place coconut oil and pumpkin puree over medium low heat.

2. Stir in the spices. Add vanilla, honey, and the coconut milk. Warm through.

3. Divide the latte between 2 cups. Sprinkle with cinnamon to serve.

Alkaline Broth

A great snack that is both high in antioxidants and anti-inflammatory nutrients. You can follow the recipe below or just keep scraps from cooking in a container in the fridge and make a broth every week. Try other herbs and other veggies because you just can't miss.

1 cup chopped beets
1 cup chopped carrots
1 cup chopped celery (optional, it is a
*   nervine and will be relaxing)*
3 medium sweet potatoes, skin on

1/2 cup cabbage
1/2 cup dark green leafy greens
Fresh herbs to taste (rosemary, thyme,
*   fennel)*

1. Place 2 quarts of filtered water to a six-quart pan.

2. Add veggies to the water. Bring to a boil with the lid on and then lower to a simmer. Simmer for 30 min and then let sit for another 30 minutes with the lid on.

3. Strain and refrigerate. Can be taken hot or cold. If you prefer hot, be careful not to boil when reheating. Make fresh as needed.

NOTE: If you don't have a sensitive GI system, you may puree the vegetables and broth together in a blender and consume as a heartier soup.

Pomegranate Lime Spritzer

A Mocktail – Pomegranate is loaded with antioxidants even in small amounts.

Grapefruit seltzer water
1 to 2 ounces of pomegranate juice
Ice cubes

1 drop of doTerra Lime Essential Oil
Lime wedges

1. Fill glass with ice and pour grapefruit seltzer three quarters of the way.
2. Fill additional one quarter of glass with pomegranate juice.
3. Squeeze one wedge of lime into the glass
4. Add 1 drop Lime essential oil and stir. Garnish with extra lime wedge.

Coconut, Cucumber, Lime & Mint Cooler

A Mocktail – Very refreshing on a hot summer evening. I find that the coconut water is sweet enough without any added sugar.

4 cups of coconut water
2 cucumbers sliced very thinly
1/2 cup of lime juice

1/4 cup of sugar (optional)
1/4 cup of chopped mint leaves

1. Combine coconut water, cucumbers, lime juice, sugar and mint leaves. Let chill for 1 to 2 hours.
2. Serve as cooler mocktails.

Citrus Basil Seltzer

A Mocktail – A tasty mocktail for the summer and not fussy to make.

1/8 wedge of a lemon
Couple leaves of basil

Plain seltzer
Couple of drops of grapefruit bitters

1. Fill a highball glass halfway with ice. Squeeze lemon over ice.
2. Muddle basil into the glass (squeeze and roll with your fingertips).
3. Fill the glass with seltzer. Add bitters and stir.

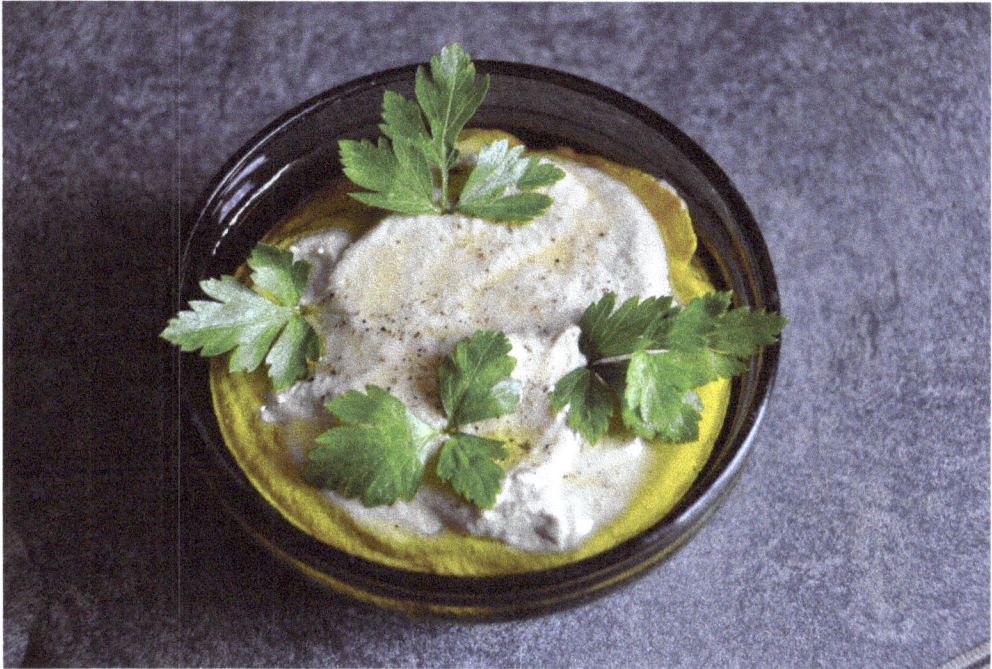

Above: Appetizers – Baba Ghanoush

Below: Appetizers – Hummus

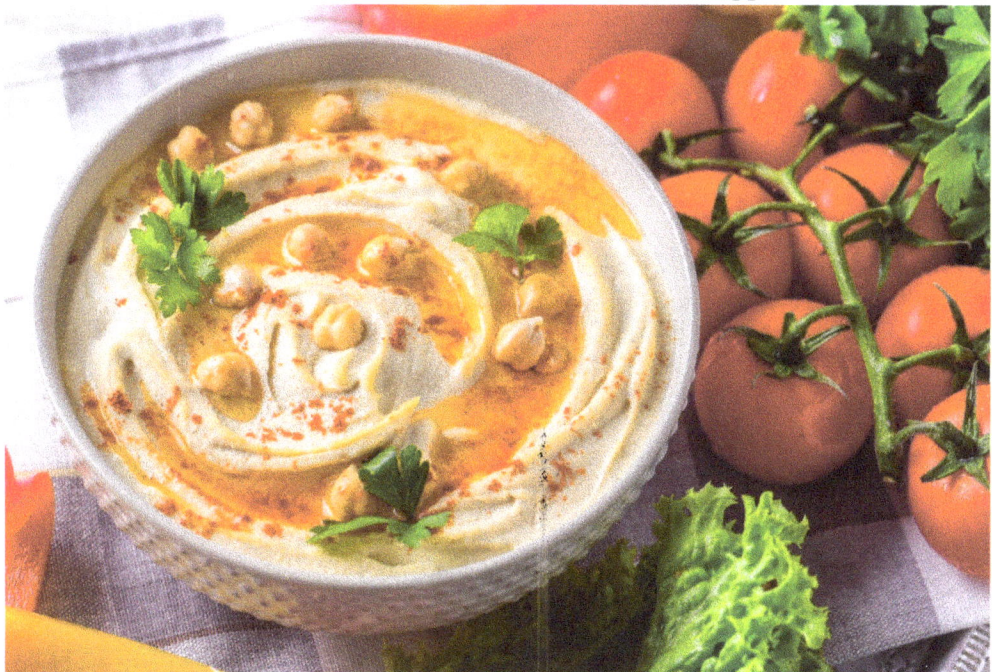

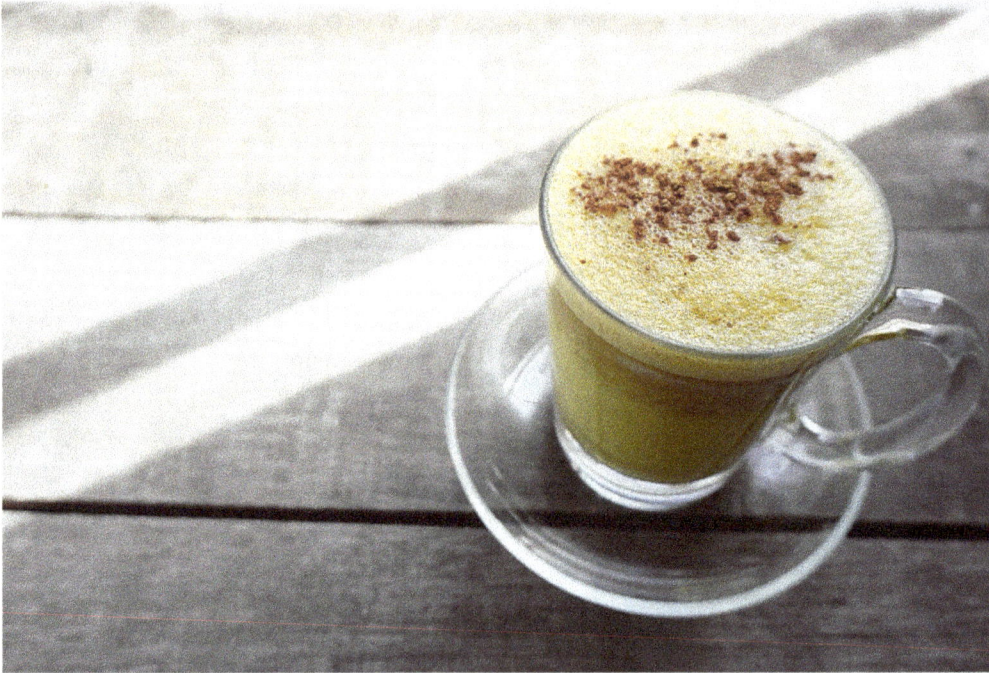

Above: Beverages – Stress-Buster Latte

Below: Beverages – Turmeric-Pumpkin Latte

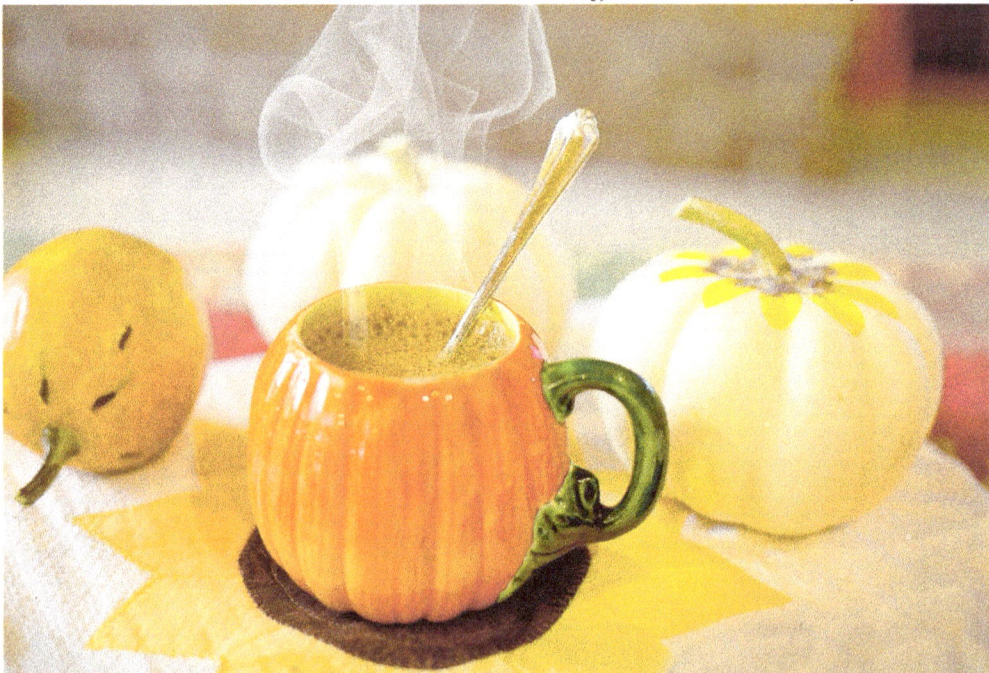

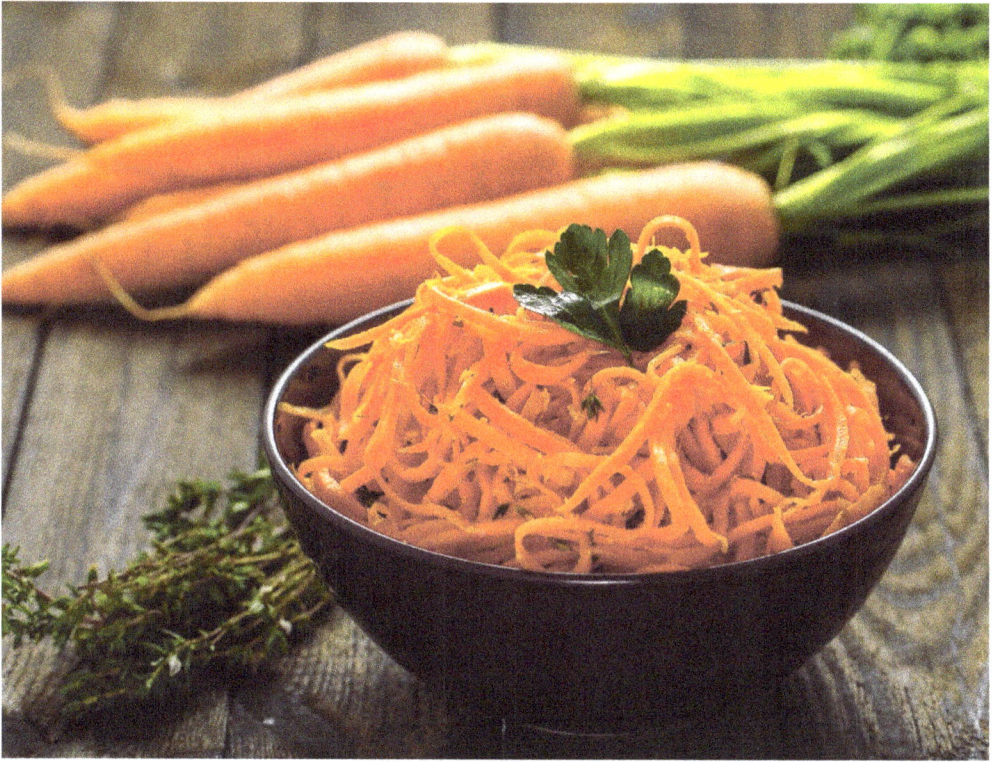

Above: Salads – Carrot Salad with Balsamic Vinegar

Below: Soups – Creamy Cauliflower Soup

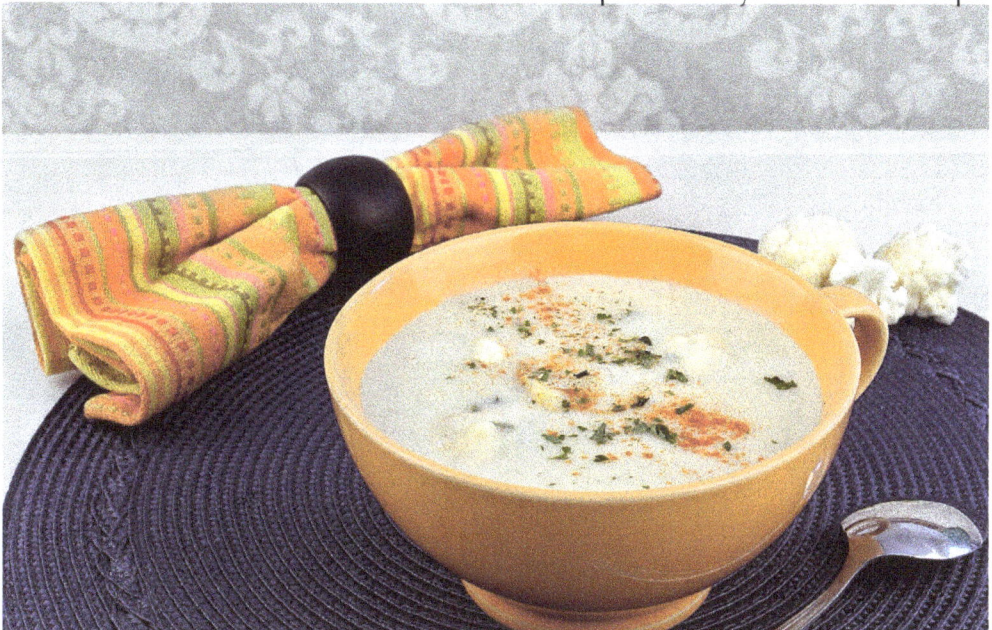

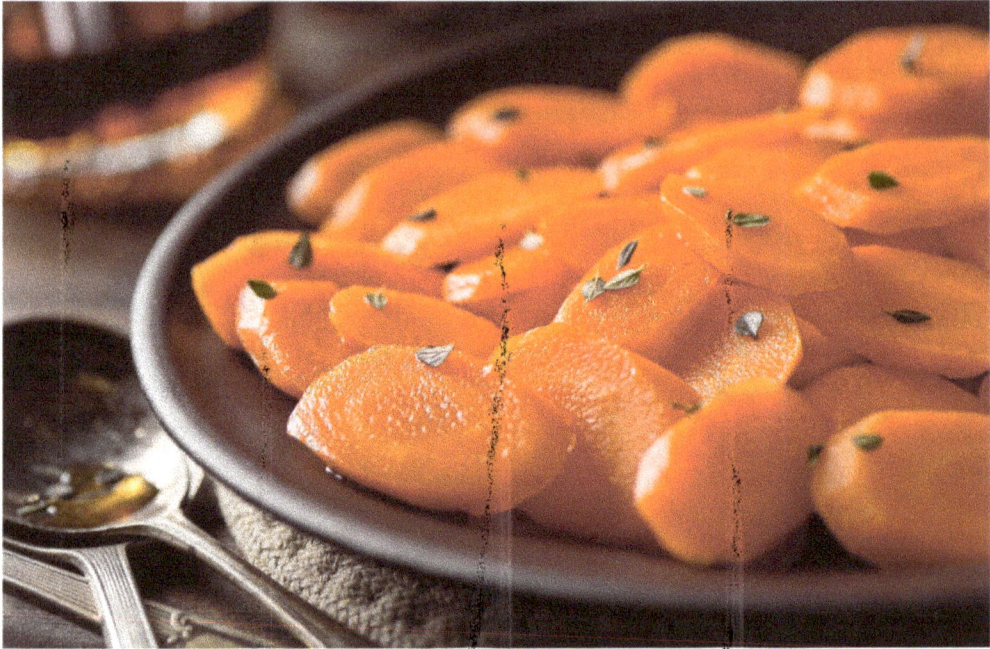

Above: Sides – Miso Glazed Carrots

Below: Sides – Roasted Summer Veggies

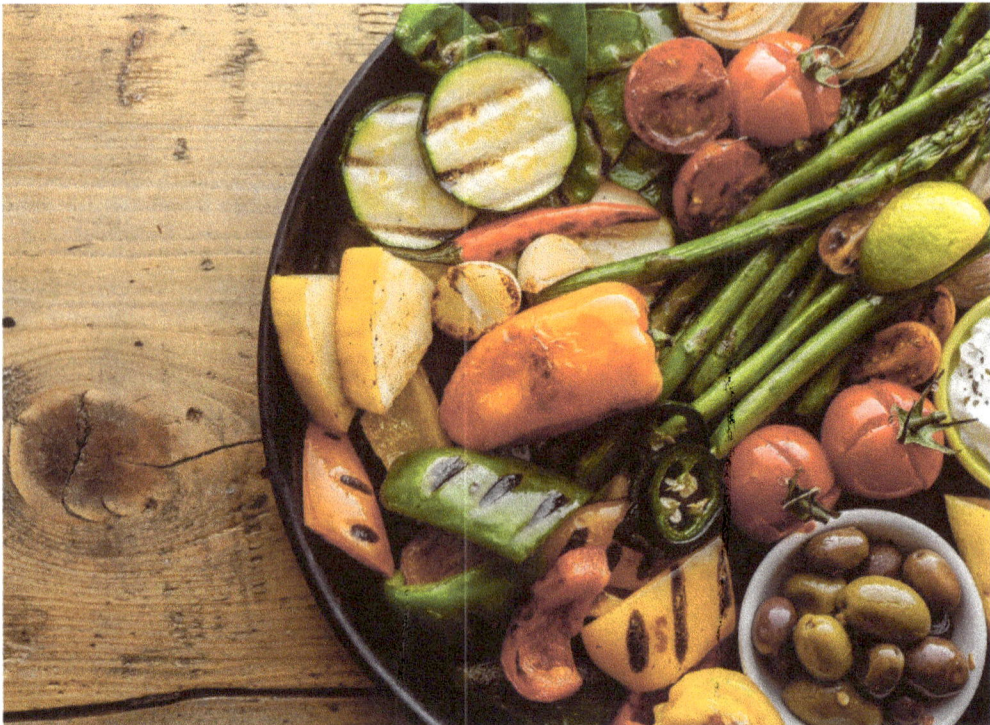

SALADS

Salads always add beautiful color to meals. Some of these salads can be used for the main course and others for side salads. Either way salads are filling while adding lots of nutrients and fiber to a meal.

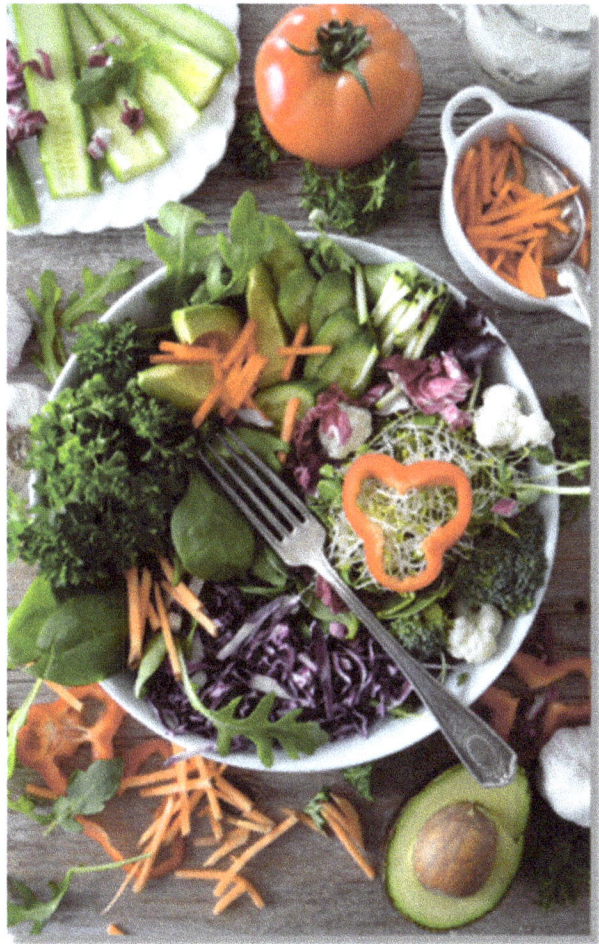

Black Bean and Quinoa Salad

A great entrée salad. Many of my clients entice their family members to try quinoa with this recipe. Quinoa is a good source of protein with 8 grams in a cup and beans are a super food in my opinion — high in fiber, nutrients and a good source of veggie protein.

1 cup quinoa
2 cups water
1/4 cup extra-virgin olive oil
2 limes, juiced
2 teaspoons ground cumin
1 teaspoon salt
1/2 teaspoon red pepper flakes, or more
   to taste

1½ cups halved cherry tomatoes
1 15-ounce can black beans, drained and
   rinsed
5 green onions, finely chopped
1/4 cup chopped fresh cilantro
Salt and ground black pepper to taste

Servings: 6-8

1. Bring quinoa and water to a boil in a saucepan. Reduce heat to medium-low, cover and simmer until quinoa is tender and water has been absorbed, 10 to 15 minutes. Set aside to cool.

2. Whisk olive oil, lime juice, cumin, 1 teaspoon salt and red pepper flakes together in a bowl.

3. Combine quinoa, tomatoes, black beans and green onions together in a bowl. Pour dressing over quinoa mixture; toss to coat.

4. Stir in cilantro; season with salt and black pepper.

5. Serve immediately or chill in refrigerator.

Carrot Salad with Balsamic Vinegar

1 carrot
2 tablespoons extra virgin olive oil
1 tablespoon balsamic vinegar
1 teaspoon honey

2 pinches salt
1 bunch parsley
1 piece garlic, grated
1 pinch pepper

Servings: 2

1. Shred the carrot and chop parsley.

2. Mix olive oil, balsamic vinegar, honey, salt, pepper, grated garlic and parsley.

3. Mix carrot and dressing.

Brussels Sprouts, Kale and Dried Cranberry Salad

I love this salad because you can make it a day ahead. This is especially helpful during the holiday season. It's colorful too!

For the Dressing:
- 1/4 cup freshly squeezed lemon juice
- 2 tablespoons pure honey
- 2 tablespoons whole grain mustard (with seeds)
- 2 tablespoons onion, minced
- 1 garlic clove, grated
- 1/2 teaspoon kosher salt
- 1/4 teaspoon freshly ground black pepper
- 1/3 cup extra virgin olive oil

For the Salad:
- 2 cups chopped kale leaves, no stems
- 2 cups thinly sliced Brussels sprouts, no stems
- 1/4 cup dried cranberries
- 1 chopped apple
- 1 cup roasted/salted almonds, roughly chopped

Servings: 6-8 as a side dish

1. Make the Dressing ahead of time: Combine all dressing ingredients in a small bowl and whisk to combine well. Add additional salt and pepper, if needed. Cover and chill.

2. In a large salad bowl, combine the kale, Brussels Sprouts, cranberries, and apples. Cover and chill until ready to serve (can be done several hours ahead of time.)

3. Up to an hour before serving, toss dressing with kale mixture until well combined. Cover and keep chilled or at room temp until serving. When ready to serve, give salad a toss again, and sprinkle with roasted almonds.

Farro Salad with Peas and Asparagus

Farro is a delicious nutty-tasting ancient grain. This is a great salad for the spring, but you can make it autumn and winter hardy by using kale, Brussels sprouts and winter squash instead of the spring vegetables and using rosemary or thyme as an herb.

1½ cups farro

12 ounces asparagus, trimmed, cut into 1
   1/2-inch lengths

1 8-ounce package peas, snow, or sugar
   snap peas

12 ounces grape tomatoes, halved

1/2 cup thinly sliced and chopped red
   onion

6 tablespoons chopped fresh dill

1/2 cup olive oil

1/4 cup Sherry wine vinegar

1 15 ounce can of chickpeas, rinsed and
   drained

1. Cook farro in large saucepan of boiling salted water until just tender, about 25 to 30 minutes. Drain. Transfer to large bowl.

2. Meanwhile, steam asparagus and sugar snap peas in another saucepan until crisp-tender, about 3 to 5 minutes. Drain. Add to farro with tomatoes, onion, and dill.

3. Whisk oil and vinegar in small bowl. Season dressing with salt and pepper. Add dressing and chickpeas to salad; toss to coat and serve.

Black Bean and Avocado Salad

For the Salad:

3 cups mixed salad greens

1 cup arugula

1/2 chopped cucumber

2 carrots, peeled and sliced

1/2 red pepper, coarsely chopped

5 to 6 scallions, slices

Healthy handful of cherry tomatoes

1 cup canned black beans, rinsed and
   drained

1/2 avocado, diced

For the Dressing:

1/4 cup extra-virgin olive oil

2 limes, juiced

2 teaspoons ground cumin

1 teaspoon salt

1/2 teaspoon red pepper flakes, or more
   to taste

2 tablespoons cilantro

Servings: 2

1. Combine greens, veggies, beans and avocado in a medium bowl.

2. For the dressing: Add all the ingredients to a jar or other airtight container. Cover and shake well.

3. Drizzle salad with dressing. Toss to combine and transfer to a large plate.

Asparagus Quinoa Salad

Serve warm as a side dish, or chilled as an Asparagus salad.

1-2 bunches asparagus
1 cup quinoa (uncooked)
1/2 cup red onion, chopped
1/2 cup kalamata olives (pitted, sliced)

1 15 ounce can of cannellini beans, rinsed
and drained
1/2 cup toasted pine nuts (optional)
Handful Italian parsley or cilantro
Zest from one lemon

Dressing:

1/3 cup olive oil
3 tablespoons whole grain mustard
2 tablespoons red wine vinegar

2 tablespoons lemon juice
1 teaspoon salt
1 teaspoon pepper

Servings: 4-6

1. Heat oven to 425° F.

2. Trim off the tough ends of the asparagus. Lay them on a baking sheet and drizzle with 1-2 tablespoons olive oil, sprinkle with a generous pinch of salt and cracked pepper, and half of the lemon zest. Roast in the oven until just tender, about 20-25 minutes. Cut into bite size pieces.

3. Bring 2 cups of salted water to a boil. Add 1 cup quinoa and cook until al dente about 20 minutes.

4. While quinoa is cooking, make the dressing. In a small bowl, stir all dressing ingredients together.

5. Place quinoa in a large bowl. Toss it with the dressing, olives, red onion, asparagus, beans, pine nuts, fresh herbs and lemon zest. Serve warm, or chill and serve as a salad.

Chicken Salad with Avocado Dressing

2 cups of cooked chicken, chopped
1/2 cup celery
1/2 cup chopped almonds or pecans
1/2 cup Avocado Dressing

Salt and pepper
Salad greens
Cherry tomatoes

1. Combine chicken, celery, nuts and avocado dressing.

2. Arrange salad greens and cherry tomatoes on a plate and mound chicken salad on top.

Fennel, Orange, Walnut and Arugula Salad

An easy fall and winter side salad. Peak growing season for fennel is fall and winter so it is a great addition to any winter salad.

1 cup walnut pieces
3 organic navel oranges
1/4 cup extra-virgin olive oil
2 tablespoons sherry vinegar or fresh
    lemon juice

Sea salt and freshly ground pepper to
    taste
1 10-ounce package of arugula
1 large fennel bulb

1. Toast walnuts in a 350° F oven for 10 minutes.

2. Grate 2 teaspoons zest from navel oranges. Whisk with oil, vinegar, salt and pepper.

3. You can either peel the oranges with a knife and section the oranges into segments, which is more elegant, or peel the oranges by hand cut in half lengthwise and slice into cross wise segments.

4. Toss arugula and fennel with dressing. Place on serving plates. Top with orange sections and toasted walnuts.

Pomegranate, Beet and Arugula Salad

This salad is beautiful. You can either use golden, red or even the Chioggia beets (red and white concentric circles) would be great. I love this hack about how to roast the beets to make them easy to peel. Pomegranate vinegar may be hard to find so just substitute either white, flavor infused or red balsamic.

2 to 3 medium sized beets
4 cups of arugula
3 tablespoons extra-virgin olive oil
1 tablespoon Pomegranate Vinegar
1 tablespoon pomegranate seeds

1/2 teaspoon sea salt
1/2 teaspoon dried thyme or 2 teaspoons
    fresh
Pinch of fresh ground pepper

1. Preheat oven to 375 °F. Wash the beets thoroughly. Wrap in aluminum foil and bake for 1 hour. Allow beets to cool. Peel the beets by rubbing with your hands covered with paper towels and cut into bite size pieces.

2. Mix olive oil, vinegar, salt, thyme & pepper together. Combine with arugula and Pomegranate seeds in a large bowl. Toss gently with beets.

No-Mayo Coleslaw

Making your own coleslaw helps to keep the sugar content low and the oil anti-inflammatory. You can substitute the lemon juice with vinegar, especially balsamic vinegar. I like fig balsamic on this. You can also purchase organic cabbage and broccoli slaw at better markets which makes this a snap to prepare.

1/4 small red cabbage
1/2 small green cabbage
1/2 carrot, shredded
Zest of 1/2 lemon
1/4 cup lemon juice

1/4 cup olive oil
1 tablespoon honey
1 teaspoon salt
1/4 teaspoon black pepper

Servings: 6-8

1. Remove any tough outer leaves from the cabbage.

2. Trim the core and any tough stems from the cabbage and thinly slice.

3. Add to a bowl with the shredded carrot, lemon zest, lemon juice, olive oil, honey, salt and black pepper. Toss to combine.

4. Serve this right away for more of a salad or store it in the fridge overnight for a slaw that's more pickled.

Citrus and Broccoli Slaw

Zesting the lime and the orange are totally worth it for this delicious side dish.

Zest and juice of 1 lime
Zest and juice of 1 orange
1½ teaspoons minced jalapeno pepper
1 teaspoon minced garlic
1/4 cup tamari
2 teaspoons maple syrup
1 tablespoon toasted sesame oil

1/2 cup red bell peppers, thinly sliced
3 tablespoons cilantro, chopped (optional)
4 cups broccoli crowns and stems, chopped in small pieces (peel stems before chopping)

Makes 4 cups

1. Make the dressing: Combine lime and orange zest and juice, jalapeno, garlic, tamari, maple syrup and sesame oil.

2. Toss dressing with the peppers, cilantro (if using), and broccoli. Serve over mixed greens or rice.

Orange, Beet and Walnut Salad

2 to 3 medium sized beets
4 cups of mixed salad greens
4 tablespoons of extra-virgin olive oil
2 tablespoons of red wine vinegar
2 oranges, peeled and cut lengthwise
    and sliced crosswise

2 tablespoons walnuts, halves or large
    pieces
1/2 teaspoon sea salt
1/2 teaspoon dried thyme or 2 teaspoons
    fresh
Pinch of fresh ground pepper

1. Preheat oven to 375° F. Wash the beets thoroughly. Wrap in aluminum foil. Bake for 1 hour. Allow beets to cool. Peel the beets by rubbing with your hands covered with paper towels and cut into bite size pieces.

2. Mix olive oil, vinegar, oranges, salt, thyme & pepper together. Combine with greens. Toss gently with beets. Sprinkle with walnuts.

Wilted Asian Salad

The cilantro, almonds, scallions and rice vinegar give this salad an Oriental flair. You can also drizzle it with toasted sesame seed oil.

1/2 head of red cabbage, thinly sliced
1 large carrot, peeled and cut into
    matchsticks
1 apple, cored, peeled and cut into
    matchsticks
4 green onions, sliced
1/2 cup chopped fresh cilantro

2 tablespoons jarred jalapeno peppers
1/2 cup roasted almonds
1 teaspoon brown sugar
3 tablespoons rice vinegar
1/4 to 1/2 teaspoon salt
1 tablespoon extra-virgin olive oil

1. In a large bowl combine cabbage, carrot, apple, green onions, cilantro, jalapeno and almonds.

2. In a small pan combine brown sugar, rice vinegar, salt and oil. Bring to a boil.

3. Pour the hot salad dressing over the veggies and toss well to combine flavors.

Mediterranean Carrot and Chickpea Salad

Thanks to my friend Linda Lindgren for this great recipe. It can be used as a side dish or a main course by just adjusting the portion size. Don't get scared off by the length of the ingredients. It's a long list of spices but they are easy to portion out. Toasting the almonds is an important step.

For the Dressing:

1/4 cup extra virgin olive oil
1 teaspoon lemon zest and
3 tablespoons lemon juice, from one
    large lemon
1/4 cup freshly squeezed orange juice,
    from one large orange
1½ tablespoons honey

3/4 teaspoon salt
1 teaspoon ground cumin
1/2 teaspoon ground ginger
1/2 teaspoon ground cinnamon
1/4 teaspoon ground coriander
1/4 teaspoon ground allspice
1/4 teaspoon cayenne pepper

For the Salad:

1 pound carrots, peeled and coarsely
    grated
1/3 cup currants
1/2 cup slivered almonds, toasted (see
    note below)
1/2 cup chopped fresh mint or cilantro
    (or mixed), plus more for serving

1 (15-ounce) can chickpeas, rinsed and
    drained
2 tablespoons finely minced shallots,
    from one large shallot
1 garlic clove, minced

Servings: 6 as side dish

1. In a large bowl (large enough to mix the entire salad), whisk together all the ingredients for the dressing.

2. To the dressing, add all the ingredients for the salad and toss well. Cover with plastic wrap and refrigerate for at least 30 minutes or up to a few hours.

3. Taste and adjust seasoning if necessary (you might need more salt, lemon or honey, depending on the sweetness of the carrots). Transfer to a serving dish and garnish with more fresh chopped herbs. Serve cold.

NOTE: To toast the almonds, preheat the oven to 350°F. Place the almonds on a foil-lined baking sheet for easy cleanup. Bake for about 5 minutes, until the almonds are golden.

White Bean and Avocado Salad

A standard salad for lunch in my household. I keep it simple by knowing we will eat this several times a week, so I make sure to keep the ingredients on hand. You can easily change it up by using a different dressing from this book or adding nuts instead of olives or avocado.

For the Salad:

3 cups mixed salad greens
1 cup arugula
1/2 chopped cucumber
2 carrots, peeled and sliced
1/2 red pepper, coarsely chopped

Handful of cherry tomatoes
1 cup canned white beans, rinsed and
   drained
1/2 avocado, diced
8 black olives, pitted

For the Dressing:

1 whole clove garlic peeled
1/4 cup red wine vinegar
1/2 cup extra-virgin olive oil
2 teaspoons chopped fresh thyme

1/4 teaspoon sea salt
1/8 teaspoon freshly ground black
   pepper

Servings: 2

1. Combine greens, veggies, beans, avocado and black olives in a medium bowl.

2. For the dressing: Smash the garlic clove with the side of a knife. Add garlic to the other ingredients in a jar or other airtight container. Cover and shake well.

3. Drizzle salad with dressing. Toss to combine and transfer to a large plate.

4. Extra dressing can be stored in the refrigerator for up to 1 week.

Healthy Cobb Salad

Traditional Cobb salad can be loaded with calories and saturated fat. This is a slimmed down version as we skip the bacon and the cheese while improving nutritional value with chickpeas, pepitas and broccoli sprouts.

For the Salad:

3 large eggs
1 cup canned chickpeas, drained, rinsed and patted dry
1/3 cup unsalted pepitas (hulled pumpkin seeds)

2 tablespoons chopped fresh chives, plus more for topping
4 cups mixed baby greens
2 ripe tomatoes, seeded and chopped
2 ounces broccoli sprouts
1/2 avocado, sliced

For Dressing:

2 tablespoons fresh lemon juice
1/4 cup extra virgin olive oil
1 tablespoon Dijon mustard

1 clove garlic peeled
1 teaspoon Salt
1/2 teaspoon fresh ground black pepper

Servings: 2

1. Place eggs in enough cool water to cover by 1 inch. Slowly bring to a boil over medium heat. When the water has reached a boil, cover and remove from heat. Let rest 12 minutes. Transfer eggs to a colander; place under cool running water to stop the cooking.

2. Make the dressing: Combine fresh lemon juice, olive oil, Dijon mustard, salt and pepper. With the broad side of the knife, lightly crush the garlic and add to dressing for at least 30 minutes.

3. Toss the greens, chickpeas, pepitas, chives, tomatoes, and avocado.

4. Peel the eggs and coarsely chop. Sprinkle on top of greens and toss with the dressing.

SOUPS

Soups are a great meal in the cooler months. They can be made ahead and easily frozen. Every time I make a soup I double or triple the recipe and add a lot more veggies than the recipe calls for. Soups are always better the second day after they are made.

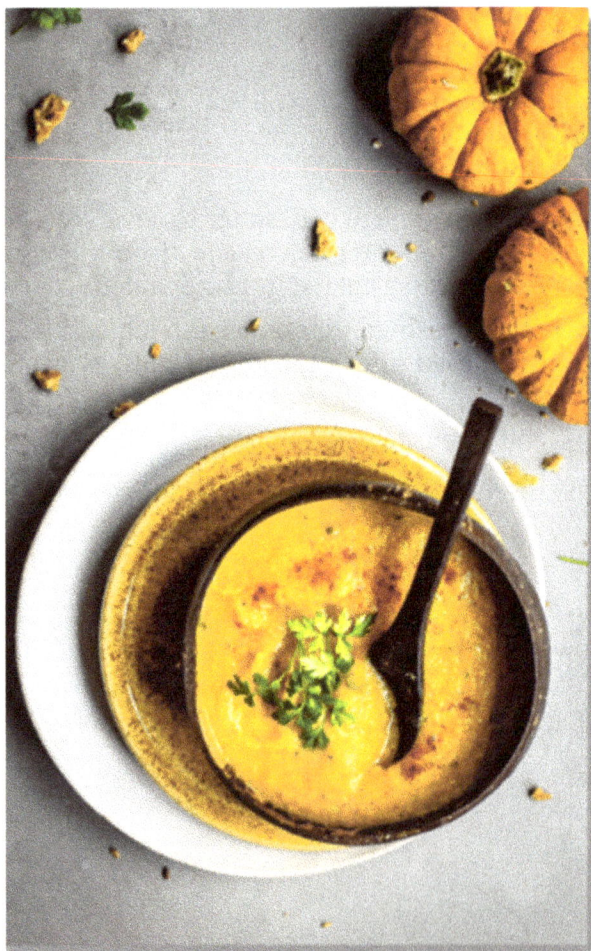

Bone Broth

See Below for Slow Cooker Bone Broth Directions

Bone Broth is a rich source of nutrients such as protein, collagen and minerals, including calcium. It is easy to use. Just add it to soups, use it in place of water when cooking vegetables, or drink it as a refreshing nourishing tea.

3½ pounds of organic beef or chicken bones (Enough bones to fill your slow cooker 3/4 of the way)
2 carrots, chopped
2 stalks of celery, chopped
2 cloves of garlic

Filtered water
1 onion
1 teaspoon sea salt
2 tablespoons apple cider vinegar
Fresh herbs such as rosemary, thyme, parsley, sage, bay leaf

1. Put the bones in a 12 quart stock pot and cover with water. Add the carrots, celery, garlic, onion, salt, vinegar and herbs.

2. Simmer 6-48 hrs. for chicken, 12 −72 hrs. for beef.

3. Strain the broth through a strainer or cheese cloth. Let the broth cool and remove the fat layer with a spoon.

Directions for Slow Cooker Bone Broth

1. Put the bones in the slow cooker.

2. Cover with cut up veggies

3. Add water to fill the slow cooker

4. Add salt, vinegar and herbs

5. Cook on low heat for 18 to 72 hours

6. Strain the broth through a strainer or cheese cloth. Let the broth cool and remove the fat layer with a spoon.

Smart Lentil Soup

I won an award for this soup at the Monadnock Wellness Festival. The ginger adds a new flavor.

2 tablespoons olive oil
1/2 pound organic gluten-free chicken
   sausage
2 cups finely chopped onion
1 cup finely chopped carrot
1 cup finely chopped celery
1 tablespoon finely minced ginger

1 to 1½ teaspoons sea salt
1 pound lentils, picked and rinsed
1 cup peeled and chopped tomatoes
2 quarts organic chicken or vegetable
   broth
1 teaspoon freshly ground coriander
1 teaspoon freshly ground toasted cumin

1. Brown sausage in a large 6-quart Dutch oven in 1 tablespoon of olive oil. Remove from pan and set aside.

2. Place the remaining olive oil into the Dutch oven and set over medium heat. Once hot, add the onion, carrot, celery and salt and sauté until the onions are translucent, approximately 6 to 7 minutes.

3. Add the lentils, tomatoes, broth, coriander and cumin and stir to combine. Increase the heat to high and bring just to a boil.

4. Reduce the heat to low, cover and cook at a low simmer until the lentils are tender, approximately 35 to 40 minutes.

5. Using a stick blender, purée to your preferred consistency. Add reserved sausage. Serve immediately.

Red Bean, Rice and Shrimp Soup

This soup is one of those great recipes that if you have a well-stocked pantry you can make this at the last minute. It's one of the reasons why I like to keep shrimp stocked in my freezer.

2 tablespoons extra-virgin olive oil
1 medium onion, chopped
4 to 6 stalks of celery, coarsely chopped
4 to 6 carrots, coarsely chopped
2 cloves garlic, minced
4 cups low sodium chicken broth
1/4 cup long-grain rice, uncooked
1 teaspoon chili powder

1/2 teaspoon cumin
1/4 teaspoon salt
1 can (14.5 ounce size) whole tomatoes (no-salt-added), undrained, chopped
3/4 pound small fresh unpeeled shrimp
1 can (15.5 ounce size) red beans, drained
1 tablespoon lime juice

1. Heat oil in a large Dutch oven over medium heat. Add onion, celery, carrot and garlic; sauté 5 minutes.

2. Add the broth and next 5 ingredients. Bring to a boil. Cover, reduce heat, and simmer for 20 minutes.

3. Peel and devein shrimp. Add shrimp and red beans to rice mixture and stir well. Cook, uncovered, 5 minutes or until shrimp is done. Remove from heat and stir in lime juice.

Chicken Vegetable Soup

1 tablespoon extra-virgin olive oil
1 small free-range chicken, cut into quarters
3 medium carrots, cut into half-moon slices

4 stalks of celery, diced
1 quart organic chicken broth
Salt and fresh ground pepper, to taste
1 cup kale or spinach
1 cup chopped fresh parsley

Servings: 4

1. Heat the oil in a medium pot over medium heat. Brown the chicken 2 to 3 minutes on each side. Remove and set aside.

2. Add the vegetables except the kale/spinach to the pan and cook for 5 minutes.

3. Put the chicken back in the pot, add the chicken broth, and bring to a boil. Reduce the heat to low, cover and simmer for about 45 minutes, until the chicken starts to fall off the bones.

4. Remove the bones. Skim any grease off the top with a ladle. Season with salt and pepper. Add the kale/spinach and allow to wilt. Add parsley and serve.

White Bean, Chicken Sausage and Kale Soup

An all-time favorite among my clients. Hearty, delicious and simple to make while chock full of fiber and nutrients.

2 to 3 tablespoons cold press olive oil
1/2 pound organic gluten free chicken
   sausage
1 large onion, chopped
5 to 6 carrots, chopped
4 to 5 stalks of celery, chopped
1/2 to 1 teaspoon sea salt

1/4 teaspoon pepper
Bay leaf
6 cups of organic chicken broth
1 bunch kale, stem removed and chopped
3 tablespoons garlic, chopped
2 (15 ounce) cans of cannellini beans,
   drained

1. Heat Dutch oven over medium heat. Add ½ tablespoon oil to pan. Sauté chicken sausage about 2 min. each side or approximately 8 minutes. Set aside.

2. Put the remainder of the oil in the pan adding onion, carrots, and celery. Sauté for about 10 minutes or until the onions are translucent. Add, salt, pepper and bay leaf.

3. Add chicken broth, bring to boil, and then set on low to simmer for 20 minutes.

4. Add kale in handfuls and allow it to cook down a bit.

5. Add garlic and add cannellini beans. Enjoy!

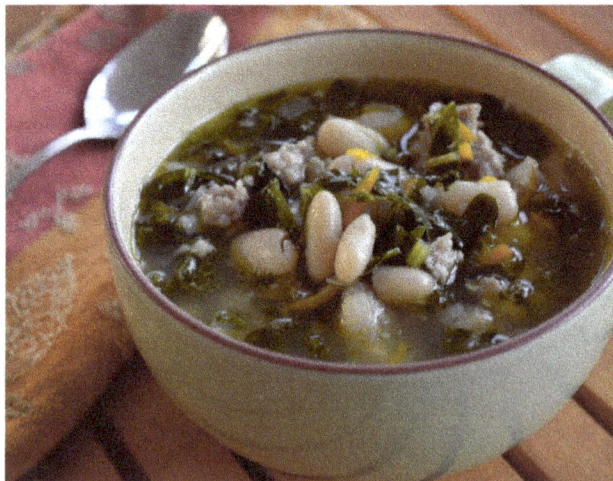

Creamy Cauliflower Soup

A great way to satisfy your desire for something creamy. Avocado does the job.

2 tablespoons olive oil
2 teaspoons chopped garlic (about 2
    cloves), plus more to taste
1 onion, chopped
Sea salt
2 teaspoons smoked paprika
1 head cauliflower, chopped
4 cups vegetable broth

1/4 cup raw unsalted cashews or 1/4 cup
    blanched slivered raw almonds
1 avocado, chopped
1 tablespoon tahini (ground sesame
    seeds)
3 tablespoons chopped chives or a
    grating of nutmeg to garnish

Servings: 4

1. In a large saucepan, heat the oil over medium heat and sauté the garlic, onions, paprika, and 1/4 teaspoon of salt for about 3 minutes, until the vegetables are soft. Add the cauliflower and sauté for another minute.

2. Add the vegetable broth, increase the heat to high and bring just to a boil. Reduce the heat to medium and simmer for about 30 minutes, until the cauliflower is completely tender. Stir the mix periodically and mash the cauliflower with a wooden spoon.

3. Remove the saucepan from the heat and allow the soup to cool slightly; stir in the nuts, avocado and tahini. Pour the soup into your blender in batches and puree on high for 1 to 2 minutes, until smooth and creamy. *

4. Return the soup to the saucepan and warm it over low heat. Stir in salt to taste. To serve, ladle the soup into bowls and garnish with either chopped chives or grated nutmeg.

*Remember to remove the plastic cap in the blender top and cover the opening with a kitchen towel so steam can escape while you blend.

Black Bean Soup

Soups are easy and I love the combination of cilantro, cumin and coriander.

2 tablespoons extra virgin olive oil, cold pressed
1 onion, chopped
1 red pepper, chopped
1 cup carrots, chopped
1 cup celery, chopped
3 cloves garlic, minced
1 cup canned crushed or whole, chopped tomatoes
1/4 cup cilantro, chopped

1 teaspoon cumin
1 teaspoon coriander
1 bay leaf
1/2 lb. gluten free chicken sausages
1½ cups vegetable stock, canned and low sodium
1/2 teaspoon salt
3 15-ounce cans of black beans, drained and rinsed
1/8 teaspoon fresh ground black pepper

1. In a large pot, heat 1 tablespoon of oil over moderate heat. Add the sausages and cook, turning until browned, about 8 minutes. Remove sausages and reserve.

2. Add the remaining 1 tablespoon oil to the pot and reduce the heat to moderately low. Add the onion and pepper. Cook stirring occasionally, until translucent, about 5 to 10 minutes. Add the garlic and cook stirring, for 30 seconds. Add the tomatoes, cilantro and bay leaf. Cook stirring frequently, for 5 minutes.

3. Slice the sausages and add to the pot along with the stock and the salt. Bring to a boil, reduce the heat, and simmer, partially covered for 15 minutes. Remove the bay leaf.

4. Meanwhile, puree 1 cup of beans and a little of the liquid from the simmering stew in a food processor or blender. Stir the pureed and whole beans and the pepper into the stew and continue cooking for 5 minutes.

5. Ladle into individual bowls and top with Greek yogurt and/or chopped parsley/cilantro.

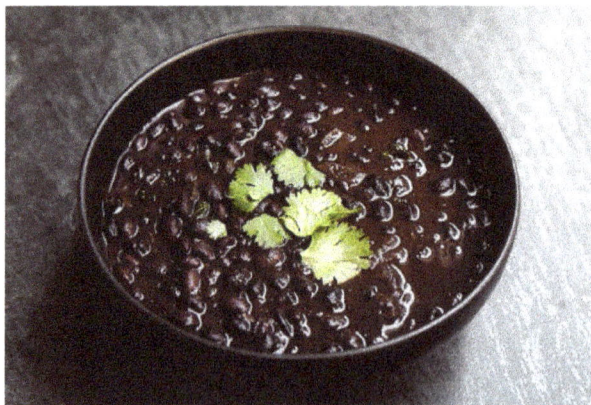

Roasted Squash and Mushroom Soup with Chicken Sausage

Wonderful soup for an autumn evening as the squash harvest is at its peak.

2 medium squash
4 cups organic chicken stock
2 tablespoons olive oil
1 onion, chopped
4 carrots, chopped
2 to 3 cloves garlic, crushed
8 ounces mushrooms, sliced
1 tablespoon diced ginger

1½ teaspoon cumin
1½ teaspoon coriander
1 teaspoon cinnamon
1/2 teaspoon mustard
1 teaspoon salt
Healthy dash of cayenne pepper
12-ounce package cooked gluten-free
    chicken sausage

1. Preheat oven 350° F. Halve and remove seeds from squash. Roast face-down in lightly oiled roasting pan for 30 minutes. Scoop out the squash when cool. Set aside.

2. On medium heat, sauté onions, ginger, garlic, mushrooms, carrots and spices for about 10 minutes.

3. Meanwhile, blend the squash and broth in blender. Add to sautéed veggies.

4. Add sausage and heat through.

Healing Mushroom Soup

A great soup for when you have a cold. Mushrooms are great for your immune system.

3 tablespoons olive oil
1 onion, thinly sliced
4 carrots, chopped
4 stalks celery, chopped
1½ pounds, assorted mushrooms,
    including shiitake and wild
    mushrooms

2 ounces dried porcini or trumpet
    mushrooms
1/2 cup hot water
6 cups organic chicken stock
Small bunch of fresh parsley
A few sprigs of fresh thyme
Salt and pepper
1/4 cup of sherry or port

1. In a medium saucepan, heat 1 1/2 tablespoon of oil over medium heat and add the onion, celery and carrot. Cook until the onion is soft and translucent.

2. Add mushrooms and remaining oil. Let the mixture cook on reduced heat for 8 to 10 minutes.

3. Stir in the chicken stock, the parsley and thyme. Bring to a boil. Reduce the heat and simmer for about an hour.

4. After an hour, remove the parsley and thyme. Let the soup cool for a few minutes. Carefully transfer about half of the mixture to the blender and blend until smooth.*

5. Return the blended mixture to the pot. Season with salt and pepper and bring to a simmer. Add the sherry or port, mix well and serve.

*The best way I have found to do this is to fill the blender no more than halfway and leave the top of the blender loosely closed. Put a dish towel over the top of the blender to keep the top of the blender from flying off and getting hot mushroom soup all over your kitchen.

Avocado Lime Soup

A great soup for the peak of the summer especially when you need to use up some avocados.

2 avocados
1 medium cucumber
1 stalk celery
Juice of 1 lime-more if you prefer
1/3 cup of cilantro
1/2 teaspoon sea salt

1 teaspoon tamari
1-2 cups organic chicken broth or veggie broth
Dairy free sour cream (see recipe below)
Chives, chopped for garnish

1. Blend all ingredients, except the sour cream and chopped chives in a high-speed blender until smooth.

2. Transfer to a serving bowl and garnish with sour cream and chopped chives.

Dairy Free Sour Cream
3/4 cup raw cashews
1 tablespoon lemon juice
2 teaspoons apple cider or sherry vinegar
1/2 cup organic chicken broth

1. Blend all ingredients in a high-speed blender. Add a little extra water 1 tablespoon at a time if you're having trouble getting the cashews smooth.

2. Transfer to a bowl or squeeze bottle and keep refrigerated. The cream will firm up a little in the refrigerator which makes an excellent dip for crudité.

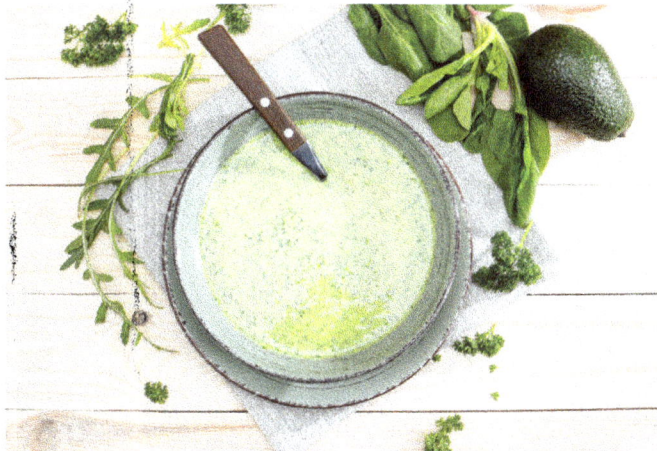

SIDES

If there is one thing all nutritionists can agree on, it's that we all need to eat more vegetables. It is worth taking the time to add flavor to your vegetables. Whether it is fresh herbs, spices, shallots, onion, nuts or garlic; if they taste good you will eat more of them!

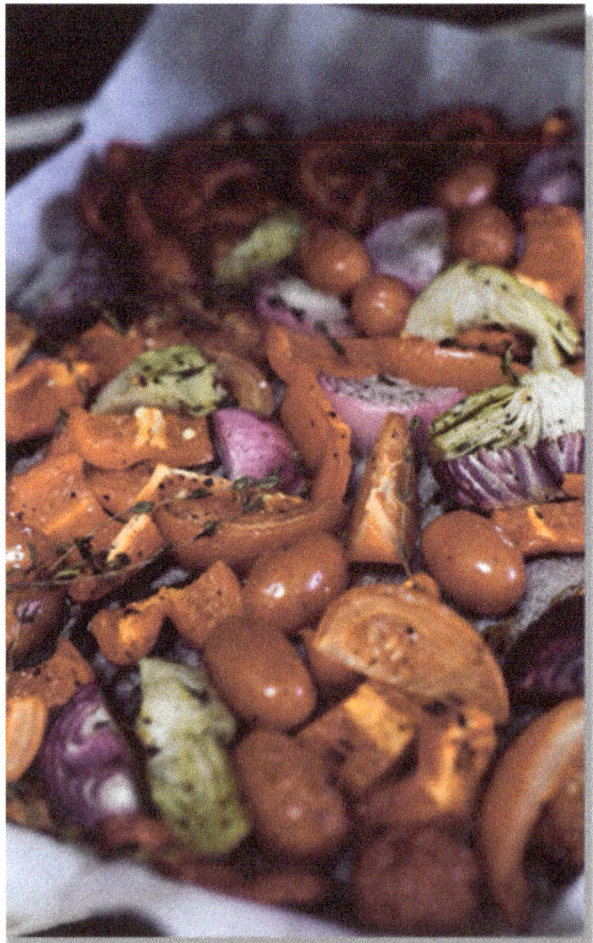

Roasted Brussels Sprouts with Balsamic Vinegar

If you aren't a fan of Brussels sprouts, you need to try this recipe. The roasting caramelizes the sprouts and the balsamic vinegar is a tasty addition.

1 pound Brussels sprouts, trimmed and halved
1 red onion, cut into wedges
2 tablespoons olive oil
Salt and pepper

1 tablespoon Penzey's* Mural of Flavor
herb mix
1 tablespoon balsamic vinegar

1. Preheat oven to 400° F.
2. Mix vegetables with olive oil, vinegar and herbs/spices
3. Roast for 20 to 30 minutes, depending on the size of sprouts.

*Check out Penzeys.com for some great herb and spice mixes and information on how to flavor food without adding excess fat and salt.

Roasted Fennel

Fennel is a totally underused vegetable. Roasting brings out its flavor.

1 large or 2 small fennel bulbs, trimmed
and cut into 1 inch pieces
2 tablespoons avocado oil
2 cloves garlic, in papery skin

1 tablespoon fresh rosemary, chopped
1 tablespoon lemon juice, fresh
1 teaspoon lemon zest
Extra virgin olive oil to drizzle

1. Preheat the oven to 400° F. Toss the fennel and garlic cloves in the avocado oil and spread on a sheet pan. Season generously with salt and pepper. Roast for 30-40 minutes, turning twice during cooking. Take out and let cool. When cool squeeze the roasted garlic out of their skins.
2. Mash the roasted fennel and garlic and combine with rosemary, lemon juice and zest. Toss and drizzle with extra-virgin olive oil.
3. Serve hot or room temperature.

Roasted Root Veggies

Great for a holiday meal or a weeknight. Make sure your herbs are fresh.

*2 large beets, peeled and cut into 1"
cubes*
*1 pound of Brussels sprouts, trimmed
and halved*
3 carrots, cut into 1" cubes
3 parsnips, cut into 1" cubes
*1 large red onion, cut in half and sliced
1/2" thick*

4-6 cloves of garlic, minced
3 tablespoons olive oil
1 tablespoon rosemary, chopped
1 tablespoon fresh sage, chopped
1/4 teaspoon salt
1/2 teaspoon pepper

1. Preheat oven to 375° F. Combine beets with 1 tablespoon oil. Spread on a large rimmed baking sheet. Roast for 30 min.

2. Combine Brussels sprouts, carrots, parsnips, onion, garlic, rosemary, sage, oil, salt and pepper in a large bowl. Split the beets between two baking sheets and add the rest of the veggies. Roast for 20 to 30 minutes.

NOTE: You can add any veggies to the roasting pan. Just bear in mind their water content. Veggies that are higher in water content like summer squash, zucchini and tomatoes don't need to roast as long. Butternut squash is a great substitute for the beets.

Roasted Summer Veggies

2 small zucchini, 1-inch pieces
2 small summer squash, 1-inch pieces
1 red onion, sliced into eighths
8 ounces quartered mushrooms
1½ tablespoons olive oil

*Penzey's Mural of Flavor seasoning or
similar*
Smoked Spanish paprika
Sea salt, pepper

Servings: 4

1. Preheat oven to 350° F.

2. Combine the squashes, red onion and mushrooms in medium baking dish.

3. Put about ½ tablespoon oil in a medium baking dish. Add vegetables and then remainder of oil. Toss to coat the veggies completely. Season with salt and pepper, Mural of Flavor, and liberal amounts of paprika.

4. Roast for 20 minutes and serve.

Spicy Cauliflower Pilaf

Spicy and anti-inflammatory.

1 head cauliflower, chopped coarsely
1 yellow onion, diced
2 tablespoons extra-virgin olive oil
1 teaspoon chili powder
1 teaspoon cumin

1 teaspoon garlic powder
1 teaspoon curry powder
1/2 teaspoon sea salt
1/4 teaspoon freshly ground black
    pepper

1. Rinse the cauliflower head and break apart into florets. Working in batches, place the florets in a food processor and process until the cauliflower begins to resemble rice.

2. In a skillet over medium heat, sauté the onion in the olive oil. When the onion become translucent, add the cauliflower to the skillet. Stir to combine and sauté the mixture until it is soft. Season with salt and seasonings to taste.

Cauliflower Mash

Another great starch alternative when you are looking for the consistency of mashed potatoes.

1 bag chopped cauliflower or 1 large
    head cauliflower, chopped
2 cups organic chicken or vegetable
    stock, plus 2 tablespoons
2 to 4 cloves of garlic, minced
Coarse salt, to taste

Freshly-ground black pepper, to taste
2 tablespoons diced fresh chives, plus
    more for garnish
2 tablespoons olive oil, plus more for
    drizzling

Servings: 4

1. Coarsely chop the cauliflower, if using. Add the chopped cauliflower and two cups stock to a medium saucepan. Bring to a boil. Turn the heat down to low and simmer for 10-15 minutes or until the cauliflower is tender.

2. While the cauliflower is cooking, heat 1 tablespoon of olive oil in a small sauté pan over medium heat and sauté the garlic until fragrant, about 30 seconds.

3. Remove the cauliflower from the pot with a slotted spoon.

4. Add the cauliflower to a food processor along with the garlic, 2 tablespoons stock, 1 tablespoon olive oil, salt and pepper. Process until combined, adding more stock if needed for desired consistency.

5. Stir in the fresh chives. Garnish with additional chives and a drizzle of olive oil.

Roasted Asparagus with Orange and Walnut

Easy but elegant vegetable dish.

4 tablespoons chopped walnuts
1½ lb. asparagus
1/4 teaspoon freshly grated orange zest

2 teaspoons fresh orange juice
1 teaspoon fresh lemon juice
2 tablespoons olive oil

1. Preheat oven to 375° F.
2. Toast walnuts in a small shallow baking pan until golden, 4 to 5 minutes. Trim woody ends from asparagus and, if desired, peel lower 2 inches of stems with a vegetable peeler.
3. Roast asparagus with 1 tablespoon olive oil on a sheet pan for about 20 minutes — more or less, depending on size of the asparagus.
4. Whisk together remaining ingredients except nuts and season with salt and freshly ground pepper to taste.
5. Transfer hot asparagus to plates. Spoon orange dressing over top and sprinkle with nuts.

Miso Glazed Carrots

Miso is fermented and a good source of soy. Great for post-menopausal vitality.

2 pounds carrots, cut diagonally into 2-
   in. lengths if large
1 teaspoon honey
2 tablespoons lemon juice
1 teaspoon grated lemon rind

2 tablespoons white miso
1 tablespoon extra-virgin olive oil
1/4 cup chopped parsley
1/2 teaspoon sea salt
2 teaspoons toasted sesame seeds

1. Toast sesame seeds in a small pan over med heat.
2. Bring a large pot of water to a boil. Reduce heat to medium. Add carrots; simmer until just tender, 8 to 10 minutes. Drain.
3. Whisk together honey, lemon juice, rind and miso.
4. Warm the olive oil in a large nonstick skillet over medium-high heat. Add carrots and miso mixture; cook, stirring frequently, until carrots are well coated, 2 to 3 minutes. Stir in parsley and salt. Transfer to a serving platter and sprinkle with sesame seeds.

Greens with Garlic and Ginger

Use any greens you want including spinach, Swiss chard, kale, and collard greens. It's quick, easy and one of those veggies it would be wise to eat daily for your liver.

1 large bunch of greens such as Swiss
    Chard, Kale or Spinach
3 garlic cloves, minced
1 tablespoon minced ginger

1 tablespoon tamari
1 tablespoon avocado oil
1/2 teaspoon sesame oil

1. Wash and chop greens into bite size pieces.

2. Heat the avocado oil in a large pan or wok at medium high heat. Add the greens and stir fry for several minutes or until wilted.

3. Add the ginger and garlic and sauté for 30 seconds.

4. Add the tamari and sesame oil. Serve.

Cauliflower with Indian Spices and Pistachios

1 medium head of cauliflower
2 tablespoons extra-virgin olive oil
3 cloves garlic, minced
1½ teaspoon ground turmeric
1 tablespoon and 1 teaspoon curry
    powder

1½ teaspoon ground cinnamon
1/2 teaspoon sea salt
3/4 teaspoon cayenne pepper
1 tablespoon lemon juice
1/4 cup pistachios, shelled

1. In a medium saucepan with a tight-fitting lid, bring to a boil 1/2 to 3/4 inch of water. Place the whole head of cauliflower in the boiling liquid, stem-side down, and cover with the lid. Reduce the heat to simmer and cook for 10 to 12 minutes, until the cauliflower is easily pierced with a knife. Remove the cauliflower from the pot and place in a shallow bowl.

2. In a small saucepan place olive oil, garlic, turmeric, curry powder, cinnamon, salt and pepper and sauté over medium heat for 3 minutes.

3. Remove from heat. Add lemon juice and pour over the steamed cauliflower. Sprinkle with shelled pistachios nuts. Serve in wedges.

Roasted Sweet Potatoes, Squash and Arugula

4 cups sweet potatoes, cubed (about 4
    medium potatoes)
4 cups butternut squash, cubed (about
    2½ pounds of squash)
2 tablespoons avocado oil
2 tablespoons balsamic vinegar

1 tablespoon fresh rosemary
3/4 teaspoon sea salt
freshly ground pepper to taste
4 cups arugula
1/4 cup pumpkin seeds

For drizzle:
Extra-virgin olive oil
Balsamic vinegar

1. Preheat oven to 400° F.
2. Toss sweet potato and butternut squash cubes with oil, rosemary, vinegar, salt, and pepper. Spread out vegetables into a single layer on 2 rimmed baking sheets.
3. Roast for about 45 minutes or until golden brown and tender, turning vegetables every 15 minutes.
4. Remove from the oven and let cool for 2-3 minutes. Toss vegetables with greens and drizzle with some additional olive oil and balsamic vinegar dressing to taste.
5. Garnish with pumpkin seeds. Serve and enjoy!

Tasty Cauliflower Rice

This cauliflower rice recipe features fresh Mediterranean flavors, including toasted almonds, lemon and parsley. It's the perfect light side dish! It's low carb, vegan and gluten free, too. You will not miss rice.

1 16-ounce bag of cauliflower rice
1/2 cup sliced almonds
1-2 tablespoons extra-virgin olive oil
2 cloves garlic, minced
Pinch of red pepper flakes
1/4 teaspoon fine sea salt

1/2 cup chopped flat-leaf parsley
1 tablespoon lemon juice
Freshly ground black pepper, to taste
Other spices to taste: smoked paprika, cumin, or curry

Servings: 4

1. Toast the almonds in the oven at 350° F. for 5 min. Reserve the almonds in a small bowl.

2. In a large skillet over medium heat, add the olive oil.

3. Once the oil is hot, add the garlic and sauté for 20 to 30 seconds. Add the cauliflower rice, red pepper flakes and salt, and stir to combine. Stir every minute or so, until the cauliflower rice is hot and turning golden in places, about 6 to 10 minutes.

4. Remove the skillet from the heat. Stir in the toasted almonds, parsley and lemon juice. Season to taste with salt and pepper and serve warm.

Roasted Garlicky Green Beans

1 lb. green beans
1 cup cherry tomatoes

1 tablespoon olive oil
2 cloves garlic minced

1. Preheat oven to 450°F. Toss green beans and tomatoes with olive oil on large rimmed baking sheet.

2. Roast until browned and almost tender, stirring occasionally, about 10 minutes. Sprinkle beans with garlic, salt, and pepper; toss to combine.

3. Continue roasting until beans are tender, about 2 minutes longer. Transfer to bowl.

Fermented Ginger-Shredded Carrots

1 tablespoon sea salt
2 cups of filtered water
4 cups grated carrots from 4– 5 medium carrots, washed but not scrubbed or peeled
1 tablespoon grated fresh ginger
1 or 2 cabbage leaves

1. Combine sea salt and water in a quart mason jar and mix until salt is completely dissolved. Set aside.

2. Grate carrots and measure out 4 cups of grated carrots. Add grated ginger to carrots and place into fermentation jar. Press down firmly to pack down into jar and remove any air bubbles.

3. Pour prepared salt brine over carrots until water level is just above the level of the carrots. Gently tap jar on the counter to remove any trapped air bubbles. Be sure to leave room in the jar as the carrots will release more liquid. Add the cabbage leaves to keep the carrots submerged in the brine.

4. Screw the lid back onto the jar and allow the jar to sit at room temperature (70° F). Set the jar on a plate away from sunlight and heat. It should take about 3 days in a warm kitchen and a day or two longer in a cool kitchen.

5. Try the carrots at day 3 and see if you like their texture and sourness. If not, let them go another day and check again. Once the ferment is the texture and taste you like transfer to the fridge and enjoy.

Fermented Carrots

1 lb. carrots, washed but not scrubbed or peeled and cut into sticks of similar size—about
*   an inch shorter than mason jar*
1 tablespoon fine sea salt
2 cups filtered water
1 to 2 cabbage leaves

Flavorings:
You can add many different herbs and spices
*   Lemon zest*
*   Dill seed*
*   Fresh Dill*
*   Garlic, peeled and smashed*
*   Chopped chives*
*   Thinly sliced ginger*

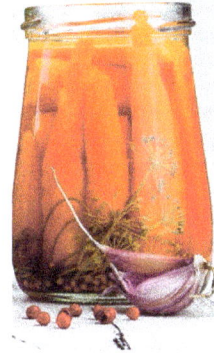

1. Sanitize a quart size mason jar and lid.

2. Place your choice(es) of flavorings in the mason jar. In a separate container add the salt to the filtered water.

3. Pack carrot sticks, standing on end, into the jar as tightly as you can. This will help prevent them from floating up the surface.

4. Pour the brined water over the carrots. Fold a cabbage leaf or 2 on top of the carrots so the carrots will be held down under the brine.

5. Screw the lid back onto the jar and allow the jar to sit at room temperature (70° F). Keep the jar away from sunlight and heat. It should take about 3 days in a warm kitchen and a day or two longer in a cool kitchen.

6. Try the carrots at day 3 and see if you like their texture and sourness. If not, let them go another day and check again. Once the ferment is the texture and taste you like transfer to the fridge and enjoy.

SAUCES & DRESSINGS

So many people think that if it is healthy, it must be bland. No way! Try these sauce recipes to amplify the flavor of your food.

Use dressings to add variety to your meals. Don't just use them on salads. They are great drizzled over veggies and add good healthy fat. You might always try to have a couple of homemade dressings around.

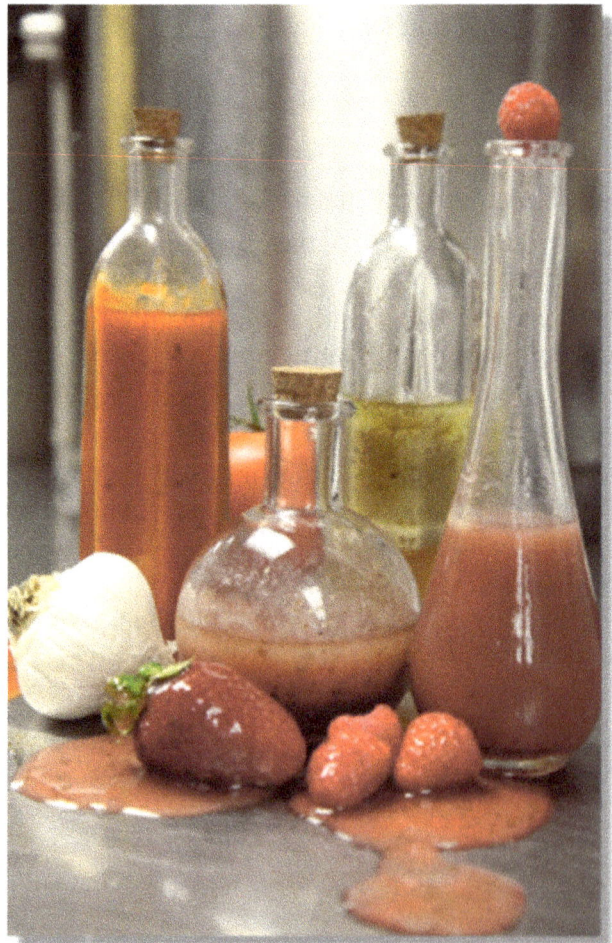

Sausage Seasoning Blend

This blend is not just for sausages, you can also add it into ground beef or turkey, or even use it for other meats, like chicken. The key ingredient (I believe) is the fennel. This gives it its distinct taste and it's delicious. Provides great flavor without the saturated fat of sausages.

First, you need to have an Italian Herbs blend, which you can buy, but it's easy to make as well. All you need to do is to mix equal parts of the base shown below and optionally customize to your taste.

Italian Herbs Blend

Mix in equal parts:

Rosemary.
Thyme
Oregano
Basil
Marjoram

To this base you can add other herbs, such as: Sage, dried Garlic, parsley.
Mix thoroughly and store in a spice jar

Sausage Seasoning Blend

2 tablespoons Italian Herbs blend (above)
3 tablespoons dried parsley
1½ tablespoon fennel seeds
1 tablespoon garlic powder

3 tablespoons salt
4 teaspoons paprika powder
4 teaspoons chili flakes
2 teaspoons sage

Put all spices in a food processor and pulse them a few times. This will break up some of the fennel seeds for extra flavor. Store in an air-tight spice jar.

Chimichurri Sauce

Developed in Argentina, this sauce is designed to be served with grilled grass fed beef. It is also great on poultry and meaty fish such as swordfish and tuna.

1 cup (packed) fresh Italian parsley
2 garlic cloves, peeled
1 tablespoon chopped fresh oregano
1/2 cup olive oil

2 tablespoons red wine vinegar
3/4 teaspoon dried crushed red pepper
1/2 teaspoon salt

1. Place parsley, garlic and oregano in a food processor. Pulse until finely chopped.
2. Transfer to a small bowl and add oil, vinegar, crushed red pepper and salt and stir until blended.

Veggie Sauce with Miso

This is a great sauce to amplify the flavor of green leafy vegetables and get some added protein and healthy fat. It's an easy way to turn veggies into a vegan entrée.

2 tablespoons fermented white miso
1½ inch piece of ginger, well washed, peeled and coarsely chopped
2 cloves of garlic, crushed
1 cup of smooth almond butter
1 tablespoon of fresh lemon juice

1 tablespoon local raw honey
1 teaspoon smoked paprika
1 teaspoon turmeric
1/8 teaspoon cayenne pepper
Sea salt and fresh ground pepper

Pulse ginger in a food processor until finely chopped. Add almond butter, miso, garlic, lemon juice, honey, paprika, turmeric, cayenne and 1/4 cup cold water and pulse. Add more water by the tablespoon to thin, if needed.

Avocado Dressing

This dressing can double as an alternative for mayonnaise.

1 medium avocado
1-2 tablespoons fresh lime juice
2-3 tablespoons olive oil

1/2 teaspoon minced garlic or shallot
1/2 teaspoon ground cumin
Sea salt to taste

Mash avocado until smooth. Add lime juice, oil garlic/shallots and ground cumin. Add sea salt to taste.

Dairy Free Pesto

It's easy to change the flavors in this basic sauce which can be used on veggies (especially spiralized), and lean meats and poultry. Choose different greens, or a variety of greens, and change up the nuts and the acid used in the recipe. Store the sauce in an airtight jar for 2 weeks, if you can keep it around that long.

2 garlic cloves, peeled
2 cups greens, lightly packed*
3 tablespoons nuts, lightly toasted—pine nuts, almonds, cashews or walnuts are great choices
1 tablespoon lemon juice

1 teaspoon lemon rind
1/2 teaspoon sea salt
Freshly ground pepper
2 tablespoons nutritional yeast flakes (optional)
3 tablespoons extra virgin olive oil

1. Place garlic, greens, nuts, lemon juice, lemon rind, salt and pepper in a food processor. If you are using the nutritional yeast flakes you can add them now. They will add a smoky cheesy flavor to the pesto.

2. Gradually add the extra-virgin olive oil in a slow stream. Taste for seasoning.

*Basil, parsley, cilantro and arugula are good choices for greens. When you use cilantro, I suggest substituting lime juice and rind for the lemon juice and rind. Arugula can easily stand up to more acid so try a tablespoon of sherry vinegar in addition to the lemon juice.

Cashew Dip

For when you have a hankering for a creamy cheese dip and dairy is not on your can-have list. It is also a great substitute for sour cream on black bean soup or chili.

1½ cups cashews
2 tablespoons lemon juice
1 tablespoon + 1 teaspoon sherry vinegar

1 cup water or chicken or vegetable broth
1/2 teaspoon salt

1. Blend all ingredients in a high-speed blender. Add a little extra water one tablespoon at a time if you're having trouble getting the cashews smooth.

2. Transfer to a serving bowl.

NOTE: This dip will firm up a little in the fridge which makes an excellent dip for crudités. Or, you can use it as a non-dairy topping for soup such as Borscht, Gazpacho or Raw Avocado Lime Soup.

Sesame Miso Vinaigrette

A great dressing for post-menopausal vitality. Sesame and miso are good for estrogen deficiency.

1 teaspoon toasted sesame seeds
1/4 cup avocado oil
1 clove garlic, crushed
2 tablespoons fresh lime juice
2 tablespoons fermented white miso

1 tablespoon tamari
1 tablespoon unseasoned rice vinegar
1 teaspoon toasted sesame oil
1/2 teaspoon grated peeled ginger

1. In a small pan toast sesame seeds over medium-high heat.
2. Mix all ingredients in a small bowl.

Champagne Vinaigrette Dressing

1 whole clove garlic, peeled and minced
1 teaspoon Dijon mustard
1/4 teaspoon sea salt

1/8 teaspoon freshly ground black
  pepper
1/4 cup champagne vinegar
1/2 cup extra-virgin olive oil

1. Combine the garlic, mustard, salt, pepper and vinegar.
2. Slowly whisk in the extra-virgin olive oil with a wire whip until emulsified.

Dijon Salad Dressing

2 tablespoons fresh lemon juice
1/4 cup extra virgin olive oil.
1 tablespoon Dijon mustard

1 clove garlic peeled
1 teaspoon salt
1/2 teaspoon fresh ground black pepper

Combine fresh lemon juice, olive oil, Dijon mustard, salt and pepper. With the broad side of the knife, lightly crush the garlic and add to dressing. Let marinate for at least 30 minutes.

Tomatillo Salsa

Great as a dip for a healthy chip or use it as a sauce for chicken and pork tenderloin.

5 medium tomatillos
1/4 cup water
1 tablespoon chopped jarred jalapeno
    pepper, seeded
handful chopped cilantro

1/4 cup finely chopped onion
1 tablespoon lime juice
1/4 teaspoon cumin
1/4 teaspoon salt

1. Peel and wash the tomatillos.
2. Place the tomatillos under a broiler for about 4 minutes each side.
3. Transfer the blackened tomatillos, and any juices from the pan to a blender or food processor. Simply add the rest of the ingredients and blend.

Tahini

Use it as a dip for veggies, a dressing, or a sauce for meat.

2 cloves of garlic, crushed
2 tablespoons fresh cilantro
2 tablespoons fresh parsley
1/2 teaspoon ground cumin
1/2 teaspoon ground fenugreek
    (optional, but good for blood sugar)

1/2 teaspoon sea salt
1/2 cup tahini
1/4 cup fresh lemon juice
1/4 cup extra-virgin olive oil

1. Pulse garlic, cilantro, parsley, cumin, fenugreek and salt in a food processor until similar in texture to pesto. Add tahini and lemon juice.
2. Slowly add oil and a small amount of water to get desired consistency.

Simple Easy Salad Dressing

1 whole clove garlic, peeled
1/4 cup balsamic vinegar, or lemon
    juice, red wine vinegar, flavored
    vinegar, etc.
1/2 cup extra-virgin olive oil

Fresh herbs to taste such as thyme,
    rosemary, dill, etc.
1/4 teaspoon sea salt
1/8 teaspoon freshly ground black
    pepper

Smash the garlic clove with the back of a knife. Add garlic to the other ingredients in a jar or other airtight container. Cover, shake well and serve. Store in the refrigerator for up to 1 week.

Tip: Change the acid and the herbs to change up the flavor. For example, you could use lime instead of vinegar or lemon juice, add some cumin and cilantro.

Good Seasons® Italian Dressing Knockoff

1 tablespoon garlic powder
1 tablespoon onion powder
2 tablespoons dried oregano
1 teaspoon pepper
1/4 teaspoon thyme

1 teaspoon basil
1 tablespoon dried parsley
1 tablespoon sea salt
1 teaspoon maple sugar (optional)

Mix together all dry ingredients and store in airtight container.

To make dressing, mix together in a jar or cruet: 1/4 cup vinegar, 2 tablespoons water, and 2 tablespoon dressing mix. Shake the jar to incorporate ingredients. Add 2/3 cup extra virgin olive oil. Mix well to combine.

Super Seed Topping

Seeds are so nutritious and delicious. Sprinkle then on salads, soups, veggies.

1/4 cup raw sunflower seeds
2 tablespoons sesame seeds
1 tablespoon fennel seeds
1 tablespoon pure maple syrup

1/4 cup hemp seeds
2 tablespoons chia seeds
Kosher salt

Servings: 8

1. Toast pumpkin seeds in a dry medium skillet over medium-low heat, tossing often, until golden, about 2 minutes.

2. Add sesame and fennel seeds; toast, tossing often, until golden brown, about 2 more minutes.

3. Mix in syrup. Cook, tossing often, until glossy clumps form, about 1 minute.

4. Remove from heat; stir in hemp and chia seeds. Season with salt.

5. Transfer to a parchment-lined baking sheet; let cool.

SNACKS

Snacks can help you get through a long day or might be helpful before or after a long workout. When it comes to snacks, just make sure you are truly in need. In other words, that you are hungry. If you are, go ahead and indulge but make it healthy with some protein, healthy fat and slowly absorbed carbs.

The snacks in this section fill the bill.

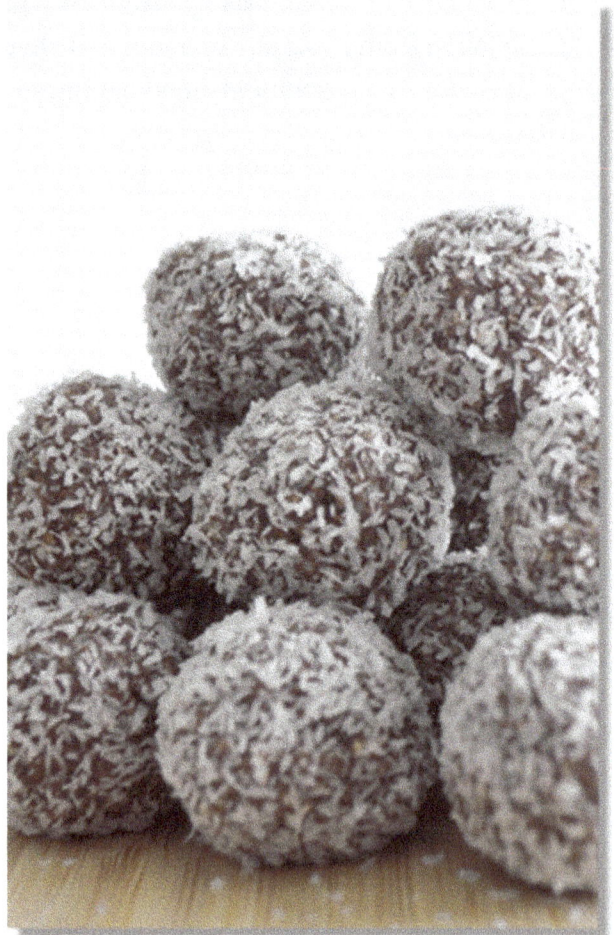

Serenity Balls

See Special Situation variations below. These are fabulous bits to keep around. You can flavor them with therapeutic herbs and essential oils to keep your hormones balanced.

Balls:

1 cup walnuts, almonds, pecans, cashews, or a mix
1/2 cup oats—gluten-free
1½ cups whole dates

2 tablespoon cacao powder
Dash of salt and vanilla, if desired
Virgin coconut oil

Coatings:

Coconut flakes
Carob powder
Cocoa powder

Sesame Seeds
Chia seeds

1. To make the balls: process the walnuts, oats and carob in your food processor until they become a rough flour.
2. Add the rest of the ingredients and process until it sticks together.
3. If it is still too crumbly or dry, add 1 tablespoon of liquid coconut oil or a few more dates.
4. Press the mix into balls (approx. 1" diameter) with your hands.
5. Roll in the coatings of your choice.

Immune Boosting Balls — Add 1 drop of wild orange and 1 drop of clove essential oil. I recommend *do*Terra essential oil because it is certified pure therapeutic grade. Roll in chopped sunflower or pumpkin seeds.

Stress Busting Balls — Add 1 tablespoon ashwagandha powder and 1 drop lavender oil. Roll in chia seeds.

Estrogen Dominance Balls — Add 1 tablespoon of roasted dandelion root and roll in chia seeds.

Low Estrogen Balls — Add up to 1 tablespoon of gelatinized maca powder. If you are new to maca, start with ¼ teaspoon and gradually increase over time. Substitute dried prunes and apricots for some of the dates. Roll in sesame seeds or cacao powder.

To Stabilize Blood Sugar — Add ½ teaspoon cinnamon and a pinch of cayenne. Roll in chia seeds.

Gorp (aka Trail Mix)

Simple and easy snack. I have a batch made up all the time.

1 cup almonds
1 cup walnuts
1 cup pecans
1 cup cashews

1 cup sunflower seeds
1 cup pumpkin seeds
1/2 cup chopped dates
1/2 cup dried blueberries

Mix together and keep in an airtight jar. Portion is ¼ cup. This makes 28 portions. A little bit goes a long way.

Grain-Free Granola Bars

Special thanks to my good friend Robin Eichert for this great recipe.

Nuts and Goodies

2 cups nuts (almonds, pecans, walnuts, cashews, any or all in whatever combination you like)
3/4 cup of sunflower seeds
4 tablespoons pepitas
4 tablespoons finely shredded unsweetened coconut

4 tablespoons cacao nibs
4 teaspoons flax seed meal
8 tablespoons coconut milk powder (can be found at Asian markets)
1/4 teaspoon xanthan gum (found in most grocery stores)
1/4 teaspoon sea salt

"Liquid"

3/4 cup peanut butter, almond butter or cashew butter
1/4 cup honey or maple syrup
1 teaspoon vanilla

1. Heat oven to 350°F.

2. Place the nuts, seeds and other ingredients of the "goodies" into a food processor. Process to achieve a uniform consistency to taste. We tend to like it chunky.

3. Warm the nut butter on stove top, add the honey and stir until mixed, then add vanilla; stir until warm (but not hot). Then stir into blended dry nut and seed mixture.

4. Once all is blended to a consistency that holds together, spread into a 10 x 13 pan lined with parchment paper. Press down firmly and evenly into pan. Cook exactly 10 minutes at 350° F. Cool.

5. Lift parchment paper onto cutting board and cut into desired size bars. With spatula, lift out onto greased cookie sheet. Cook for another 10 minutes at 350° F. Cool and store.

Turkey Roll-Ups

A good hearty snack with good lean protein and veggies.

8 slices nitrate-free turkey
1 cup of tomato, chopped
1 cup of cucumber, chopped
1 avocado cut into eighths
Grated carrot

1. Chop up tomato and cucumber. Cut the avocado into eighths and grate the carrot.

2. Place 2 tablespoons of tomato and cucumber on the end of the slice of turkey. Add the avocado and the carrot and roll the turkey around the filling.

Avocado Prosciutto Roll-Ups

1 avocado, cut in eighths
8 slices prosciutto
2 tablespoons extra-virgin olive oil
1 tablespoon fresh lemon juice
Sea salt and freshly ground black pepper

1. Wrap each avocado slice with a slice of prosciutto. Sprinkle with olive oil, lemon juice, salt and pepper.

2. Sprinkle with seasonal herbs such as dill in the spring, basil in the summer, and thyme in the fall.

Almond Butter Balls

Great for those moments when you would like something sweet but want to stay on the healthy side.

1 cup almond butter
2/3 cup dates
2 teaspoons vanilla extract
2 cups gluten free old-fashioned rolled oats

2 cups shredded unsweetened coconut
1 cup ground flaxseed
1 cup mini dark chocolate chips
1/2 cup dried cherries

1. Mix almond butter, honey and vanilla extract together thoroughly.
2. Add all the rest of the ingredients and mix well in food processor.
3. Using a heaping tablespoon create bite-sized pieces.
4. Refrigerate and store in an air-tight container.

Roasted Nuts with Herbs

These nuts are simple to make and always get rave reviews. Just make sure your oven temperature is only 200 degrees. It is worth buying an inexpensive oven thermometer to be sure. And make sure you start with raw nuts. A perfect recipe for the holidays because they are so easy.

4 cups mixed raw nuts, such as walnuts, cashews, pecans and almonds
32 fresh sage leaves, torn into large pieces

One 8-inch fresh rosemary sprig
4 sprigs of fresh thyme
3 tablespoons extra-virgin olive oil
Salt and freshly ground pepper

1. Preheat oven to 200° F. No higher. This is necessary to keep the nuts from burning.
2. Using a large rimmed baking sheet, toss the nuts with the sage, rosemary, thyme and olive oil.
3. Season with salt and pepper.
4. Roast for 3 hours. Make sure they don't brown.
5. Let the nuts cool until crisp. Store in air-tight containers.

Tofu Snacks

1 Recipe of Crispy Baked Tofu, warm or room temp (see Entrees)
1 Recipe of Dipping Sauce (Recipes below)

Dip the tofu into or drizzle with Dipping Sauce for a tasty treat.

Thai Chili Dipping Sauce

1 tablespoon extra-virgin olive oil
1½ teaspoons rice vinegar
1½ tablespoons tamari, low sodium
1 teaspoon Sriracha sauce, or to taste

Mix all ingredients and dip or drizzle.

Thai of Another Flavor Dipping Sauce

1/4 cup chicken stock
1 tablespoon black bean sauce
1½ teaspoons roasted red chili paste
1 teaspoon tamari, low sodium
1/2 teaspoon honey
1/4 teaspoon garlic powder

Mix all ingredients and dip or drizzle.

Orange Sesame Dipping Sauce

2 tablespoons tamari, low sodium
1 tablespoon fish sauce
2 tablespoons fresh orange juice
1½ teaspoons orange zest
2 teaspoons sesame oil
1 teaspoon honey

Mix all ingredients and dip or drizzle.

ENTREES

Most of the recipes in this section can be made in 20 to 30 minutes. A few take longer but are perfect for a weekend afternoon

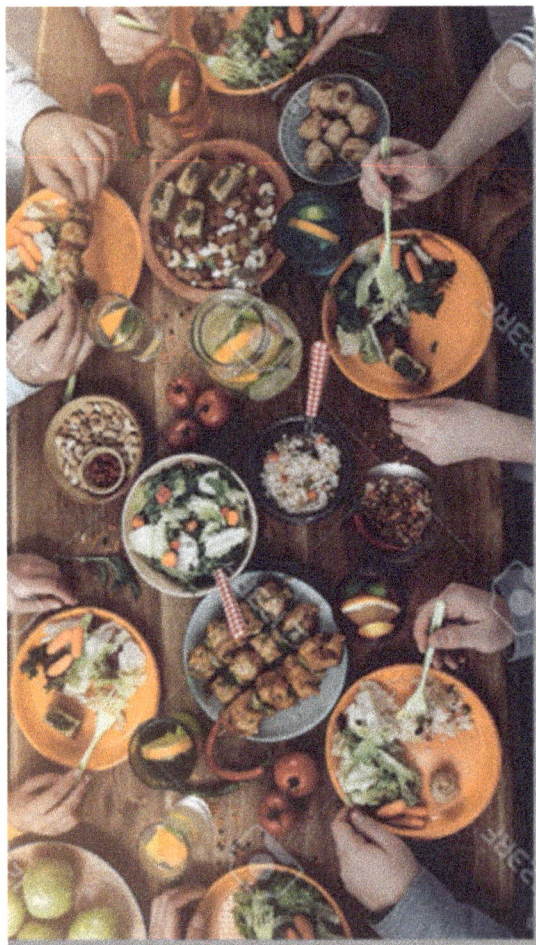

Smoky Paprika Baked Chicken Breast

This a simple, easy and delicious chicken recipe. The smoked paprika makes it very flavorful, moist and quick.

4 6-ounce organic chicken breasts
2 tablespoons olive oil

Smoked Spanish paprika
Sea salt, pepper

Servings: 4

1. Preheat oven to 350° F.

2. Put about ½ tablespoon oil in a medium baking dish. Coat both sides of the chicken breast. Season the chicken with salt and pepper and liberal amounts of paprika.

3. Roast for about 20 minutes and serve with roasted mixed vegetables.

Tandoori Chicken

The chicken is poached so you can make it ahead if you want. All the spices work together to make it spicy but not hot.

2 pounds chicken breasts, fat trimmed and cut into palm-sized portions
4 cups organic chicken stock
1/2 onion, chopped finely
2 cloves garlic, minced
Pinch sea salt
1/2 cup full fat or reduced fat coconut milk

1 teaspoon sea salt
1 teaspoon smoked paprika
1/2 teaspoon cayenne pepper
1 teaspoon cumin
1 teaspoon coriander
1/2 teaspoon garlic powder
1 teaspoon turmeric
1 teaspoon black pepper

Servings: 6

1. Fill a large pot with chicken stock and add the garlic and onion. Bring to a boil.

2. Once boiling, add the chicken breasts and reduce to low and simmer for 12-15 minutes, until chicken is just cooked and no longer pink. Remove from heat and drain immediately and allow chicken to cool. You can save the broth for other purposes.

3. Set the chicken aside to cool.

4. Combine all the spices in a small bowl and add the coconut milk. Mix until combined.

5. Once cooled, place chicken back into the pot and using two forks, shred the chicken finely. Add the sauce and serve immediately.

Sautéed Chicken with Olives, Capers and Lemons

2 lemons, sliced ¼-inch thick
1/4 cup plus 1 tablespoon extra-virgin
    olive oil
6 skinless, boneless chicken thighs, about
    1 pound
1-2 tablespoons brown rice flour
1 fat garlic clove, minced

1 cup organic chicken broth
3/4 cup Sicilian green olives
1/4 cup capers
2 tablespoons parsley
Kosher salt and freshly cracked black
    pepper

Servings: 4

1. Bring a medium-large, high sided skillet to medium-high heat and add 1 tablespoon of olive oil. Add half of the lemon slices and sear until browned, 3-5 minutes on each side. Transfer to a plate.

2. Season the chicken thighs with kosher salt and black pepper and dust with rice flour, shaking off the excess. Add 1½ tablespoons of olive oil to the hot pan and sear the chicken pieces until golden brown, about 5 minutes each side. Transfer to another plate and finish searing the rest of the chicken pieces and add to the rest of the chicken.

3. Add the rest of the olive oil to the pan and the minced garlic and cook for 30 seconds or until fragrant. Add the green olives, capers and broth. Add the reserved chicken and any juices that have been released plus the reserved lemons and their juices and cook over high heat until the broth is reduced by half, about 5 minutes. Add parsley and cook for another minute. Season with more kosher salt and freshly ground black pepper to taste.

4. Transfer to plates and spoon the olives, capers, lemons and sauce on top. Serve with sautéed spinach, kale or Swiss chard on the side.

Roasted Veggies & Chicken Sausage

I love this recipe because it is so easy to make and to clean up after.

2 large beets, peeled and cut into 1-inch cubes
1 pound of Brussels sprouts, trimmed and halved
3 carrots, cut into 1-inch cubes
3 parsnips, cut into 1-inch cubes
1 large red onion, cut in half and sliced ½-inch thick

4-6 cloves of garlic, minced
3 tablespoons olive oil
1 tablespoon rosemary, chopped
1 tablespoon fresh sage, chopped
1/4 teaspoon salt
1/2 teaspoon pepper
4 links cooked chicken sausage, gluten-free

Servings: 4

1. Preheat oven to 375° F. Combine beets with 1 tablespoon oil. Spread on a large rimmed baking sheet. Roast for 15 minutes.

2. Combine Brussels sprouts, carrots, parsnips, onion, garlic, rosemary, sage, oil, salt and pepper in a large bowl. Split the beets between two baking sheets and add the rest of the veggies. Roast for 10 minutes.

3. Stir the veggies and place sausages on the pan. Continue roasting, stirring once or twice or until veggies are tender, about 20 minutes more.

NOTE: You can add any veggies to the roasting pan. Just bear in mind their water content. Veggies that are higher in water content like summer squash, zucchini and tomatoes don't need to roast as long. Butternut squash is a great substitute for the beets.

Grilled Chicken with Garlic Pesto

4 boneless and skinless chicken breasts
2 cloves of garlic

2 tablespoons extra-virgin olive oil
2 tablespoons to 1/4 cup basil

1. Mince the garlic and combine with oil and basil.

2. Spread garlic basil mixture on the chicken breasts and let marinate for about an hour.

3. Grill or bake the chicken breasts.

Turkey Cutlets with Mushrooms & Marsala

Turkey is a great lean protein. This dish is elegant enough for a special dinner meal. And of course, mushrooms are awesome.

1¼ lb. turkey breast cutlets
Coarse salt and freshly ground pepper,
   to taste
3 tablespoons olive oil, plus additional as
   needed
1 to 2 tablespoons all-purpose flour
1 large shallot, minced

1 lb. button or cremini mushrooms,
   sliced
1 cup dry Marsala
3/4 cup low-sodium chicken broth
3 tablespoons minced fresh thyme
1 to 2 tablespoons unsalted grass-fed
   butter, clarified*

Servings: 4

1. Rinse the cutlets with cold water and pat dry with paper towels. Season the turkey cutlets on both sides with salt and pepper. Sprinkle some of the flour on a shallow plate or waxed paper.

2. Heat 1 tablespoon olive oil in a large nonstick skillet over medium-high heat. Dust about half the turkey in flour and add to the pan. Cook, turning once, until just brown, about 2 minutes per side. Put them aside and keep warm. Repeat with the remaining turkey adding 1/2 tablespoon olive oil to the pan as needed).

3. In the same pan over medium-high heat, warm the remaining 1½ tablespoon olive oil. Add the shallot and sauté until fragrant, about 30 seconds. Add the mushrooms, season lightly with salt and pepper and sauté until the mushroom juices are absorbed, about 4 minutes.

4. Add the Marsala and broth and bring to a boil. Continue at a gentle boil until the juices reduce and thicken slightly, about 8 minutes. Add the thyme and butter and stir until the butter dissolves. Return the turkey and any juices on the platter to the skillet. Simmer, turning the turkey occasionally, until the sauce thickens slightly, about 3 minutes.

5. Serve immediately. The turkey cutlets go well on quinoa or brown rice with the sauce and mushrooms ladled over both.

*To clarify butter, melt a stick of butter over medium-high heat until the mixture bubbles. Scrape the bubbles off and pour the golden liquid that remains into a bowl, leaving the white milk solids behind. Your butter is now dairy free.

Chickpea Masala

You can have this dish on the table in less than 15 minutes if you do some pre prep. Just cut up the onion, pepper and zucchini ahead of time and store in fridge.

1/2 small red onion
1 yellow bell pepper
1 medium zucchini
coconut oil or ghee
1 teaspoon garam masala*
1/2 teaspoon cumin
1/4 teaspoon turmeric

1/2 teaspoon salt, more to taste
1 14-ounce can chopped tomatoes
1 14-ounce can chickpeas, rinsed and
    drained
1 cup full-fat canned coconut milk
cilantro, to serve

Servings: 4

1. Finely chop red onion and bell pepper and cut zucchini into small, bite-size chunks.

2. Heat oil in a large pan (with a lid) over medium-high heat. Add onion and pepper and cook, stirring for 2-3 minutes until softened. Add zucchini and cook for 1 minute. Stir in garam masala, cumin, turmeric, and salt, and cook for 1 minute.

3. Stir in tomatoes and chickpeas, and cover. Cook for 5 minutes, stirring about halfway through. Uncover, stir in coconut milk, and reduce heat to medium. Cook for 2 more minutes.

4. Serve over rice, quinoa, or greens with a little chopped cilantro.

    *Garam masala is a blend of ground spices common in cuisines from India.

Eggplant, Tomato & Chickpea Stew
(Slow-Cooker)

1 onion, chopped
2 eggplants, cut into 1" cubes
2 15-oz. cans diced tomatoes, with juices
4 cloves garlic, minced

2 tablespoons finely chopped fresh
    ginger
1 tablespoon curry powder
2 teaspoons cumin
Salt and pepper

Servings: about 6

1. Combine onion, eggplant, garlic, ginger, curry, cumin, tomatoes with juices, and 1 teaspoon salt in a large slow-cooker and stir well.

2. Cover and cook on low until eggplants are soft, 5 to 6 hours.

3. Stir in chickpeas; cover and cook until warmed through, about 15 minutes longer. Season with salt and pepper and serve.

Vegetable Curry

1 sweet potato, peeled and cubed
1 medium eggplant, cubed
1 green bell pepper, chopped
1 red bell pepper, chopped
2 carrots, chopped
1 onion, chopped
5 tablespoons olive oil, cold pressed
3 cloves garlic, minced
1½ teaspoon ground turmeric
1 tablespoon and 1 teaspoon curry
   powder

1½ teaspoon ground cinnamon
1½ teaspoon salt
3/4 teaspoon cayenne pepper
1 15-ounce can garbanzo beans
1/4 cup sliced or chopped almonds
2 tablespoons raisins
1 zucchini, sliced
1 cup orange juice
10 ounces of spinach

Servings: 4 - 6

1. In a large Dutch oven place sweet potato, eggplant, peppers, carrots, onion and 2 tablespoons olive oil. Sauté for 5 minutes over medium heat.

2. In a small saucepan place 3 tablespoons of olive oil, garlic, turmeric, curry powder, cinnamon, salt and pepper and sauté over medium heat for 3 minutes.

3. Pour garlic and spice mixture into the Dutch oven with vegetables in it. Add the garbanzo beans, almonds, zucchini, raisins and orange juice. Simmer 20 minutes covered.

4. Add spinach to pot and heat for 5 more minutes. Serve with brown rice.

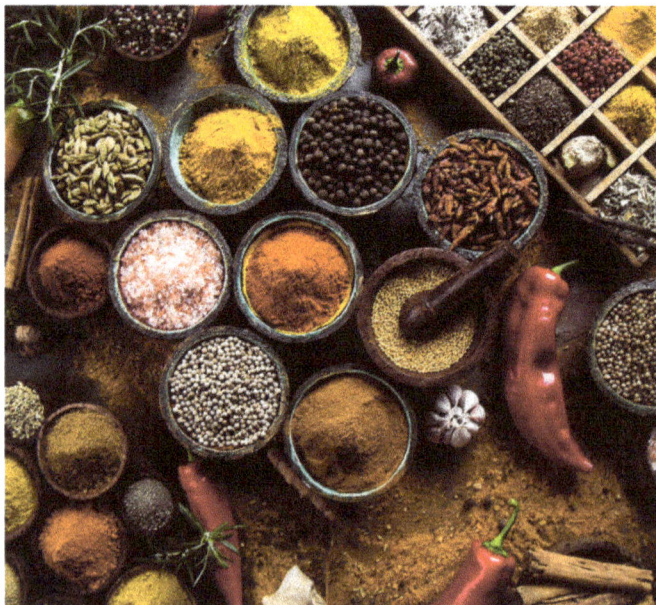

Spinach and Chickpea Curry

2 tablespoons olive oil
1/2 thinly sliced red onion
2 tablespoons finely chopped fresh
    ginger
1 or 2 cloves of garlic, finely minced
1 tablespoon curry powder
1 teaspoon garam masala

1/8 teaspoon cayenne pepper
1 15-oz. can chickpeas, rinsed and
    drained
14½ oz. can diced tomatoes
1 teaspoon salt
7 packed cups of baby spinach
1/4 cup fresh cilantro, chopped

Servings: 2

1. Heat olive oil in a sauté pan over medium heat. Add onion, ginger, garlic, curry powder, garam masala and cayenne. Cook, stirring often, until the onion is soft, about 5 minutes.

2. Stir in the chickpeas, tomatoes and salt.

3. Add the baby spinach by the handful, stirring to wilt as you go. Continue to cook until the spinach is wilted, about 5 minutes more.

4. Season to taste with salt and pepper. Remove the pan from the heat and stir in the cilantro.

5. Serve with brown rice, amaranth or quinoa.

Shrimp Curry

An easy meal to whip *up for company if you have a well-stocked pantry. You might want to keep both frozen shrimp and reduced fat coconut milk always on hand.*

1 pound uncooked, deveined shrimp
1/2 diced onion
4 cloves garlic
1/2 cup reduced fat coconut milk
1-3 whole tomatoes, chopped

2 tablespoons tomato paste
1/2 teaspoon Garam Masala seasoning
1½ teaspoon coriander
1/2 teaspoon cumin
1/2 teaspoon curry powder

Servings: 4

1. On medium-low heat, sauté onions in olive oil until translucent.

2. Add garlic, shrimp, and all the powder seasonings.

3. Let it cook for a bit, then add in some coconut milk, and the tomatoes.

4. Stir, let it continue to cook on a simmer until it thickens.

5. Then add tomato paste. Mix in well and heat thoroughly.

6. Serve with brown rice or quinoa.

Buffalo Burger on a Portabella Mushroom

A great low carb alternative to a burger on a bun. And the buffalo burger is rich but relatively low fat.

1 pound Buffalo meat, grass fed
4 Portabella mushroom caps*
1/4 cup olive oil

4 tablespoons chopped onion
4 cloves of garlic, minced
4 tablespoons balsamic vinegar

Garnish(es) of Choice: Mustard, avocado slices, grilled red onion, tomato slice, lettuce/romaine/spinach...

Servings: 4

1. Clean mushrooms and remove stems, reserve for other use. Place caps on a plate with the gills up.

2. In a small bowl, combine the oil, onion, garlic and vinegar.

3. Pour mixture evenly over the mushroom caps and let stand for 1 hour.

4. Form the Buffalo meat into 4 patties approximately the size of the mushroom caps. Season per your preferences.

5. Broil or grill the burgers 5 minutes per side and the mushrooms for 10 minutes. Serve the burgers on the mushroom caps and garnish.

*To use the caps like a bun, double the number of mushrooms and increase the onion, garlic and vinegar by about one-half. Put the caps on & take them off the grill/broiler a few minutes before the burgers to let them cool slightly.

Roast Cod with Cherry Tomatoes, Olives and Capers

One of my favorites! A simple delicious meal. It tastes great when cherry tomatoes are in season and straight out of the garden. Super colorful.

4 6- to 8-ounce pieces skinless cod
8 ounces cherry or grape tomatoes
   (about 1/2 cups)
2 tablespoons extra-virgin olive, cold-
   pressed
Sea salt
Fresh ground pepper

1/3 cup Kalamata olives
2 tablespoons capers, rinsed and soaked
   in cold water for 10 minutes
2 to 3 garlic cloves, minced
1 teaspoon fresh lemon juice
1 tablespoon clarified butter or ghee
3 tablespoons thinly sliced basil leaves

Servings: 4

1. Heat oven to 450° F with rack in middle.
2. In a large skillet arrange cod pieces. Add tomatoes, arranging them around and over the cod. Drizzle with oil and season with salt and pepper.
3. Roast until fish is opaque and tomatoes are burst, about 14 minutes.
4. If tomatoes have not burst, transfer fish to a plate and return skillet to oven for 2 or 3 more minutes.
5. Transfer fish to serving plates.
6. Sauté garlic for 30 seconds.
7. Add capers, olives and lemon juice to skillet, bring juices to a simmer over medium heat.
8. Whisk in butter.
9. Spoon juices over fish, sprinkle with basil and serve immediately.

Spicy Coconut Salmon with Bok Choy

Bok choy is a brassica vegetable, so it is high in nutrients. This dish is super easy and quick to make with the added benefit of salmon.

1 tablespoon olive oil
4 6-ounce salmon fillets
1/4 teaspoon salt
1/4 teaspoon pepper
1 red onion, thinly sliced
1/4 teaspoon cayenne pepper

*1 13.6-ounce can unsweetened light
  coconut milk*
1 tablespoon lemon juice
*1 head (1 pound) Bok choy chopped or 5
  to 6 baby Bok choy*
Fresh basil

Servings: 4

1. In a skillet, heat oil over medium high heat. Season salmon fillets with salt and pepper and cook until golden, 2 minutes per side. Transfer to a plate.

2. Cook red onion with a pinch of salt and cayenne pepper, stirring until golden, about 6 minutes. Add unsweetened light coconut milk and lemon juice. Simmer, stirring, 10 minutes.

3. Add Bok choy and simmer 1 minute. Return salmon to pan and simmer for 2 minutes.

4. Season to taste and garnish with fresh basil.

Arugula Salad with Fennel and Roasted Salmon or Cod

2 6-ounce salmon or cod filets
4 cups arugula leaves
1/2 avocado
1 bulb fennel, thinly sliced

*1 tablespoon cold-pressed extra-virgin
  olive oil*
1/2 lemon
1/2 to 1 teaspoon sea salt

Seasoning (Emeril's Original Essence or Penzey's Northwoods are good)

Servings: 2

1. Preheat oven to 350° F.

2. Combine all ingredients but salmon/cod and seasoning in a bowl and toss.

3. Brush fish with oil and season. Roast for 20 minutes.

4. Serve salad in a mound and top with salmon filet.

Spiced Salmon with Mustard Sauce

2 teaspoons whole-grain mustard
1 teaspoon honey
1/4 teaspoon ground turmeric
1/4 teaspoon ground red pepper

1/8 teaspoon garlic powder
1/4 teaspoon salt
4 (6 ounce) salmon fillets

Servings: 4

1. Preheat oven to 425° F.

2. Combine all the ingredients but the salmon in a small bowl. Rub mustard mixture over each fillet.

3. Place fillets, skin side down on a pan coated with cooking spray.

4. Cook for about 15 minutes or until fish flakes easily. Exact time will depend on how thick the fish is.

Salmon with Crispy Cabbage and Kale

1 bunch Lacinato kale, tough stems removed, leaves thinly sliced (about 2½ cups)
1/4 head Savoy cabbage, cored and thinly sliced (about 2 cups)
3 tablespoons olive oil, divided
Kosher salt
2 salmon fillets (4 to 6 ounces each)

1/4 to 1/2 teaspoon seafood seasoning (I love Paul Prudhomme's Seafood Magic)
1/2 teaspoon lemon zest plus 1 tablespoon lemon juice
2 tablespoons chopped fresh dill
1/2 teaspoon Dijon mustard

Servings: 2

1. Preheat oven to 450° F.

2. On a quarter-sheet pan, toss kale and cabbage with 1 tablespoon oil, and spread in an even layer; season with salt and bake 6 minutes. Season salmon with seafood seasoning, and add to baking sheet, skin side down. Bake until salmon is cooked through, about 8-9 minutes.

3. Meanwhile, whisk together lemon zest and juice, dill, mustard, and remaining 2 tablespoons oil. Season to taste with salt.

4. Drizzle salmon and vegetables with dressing before serving.

Sesame Encrusted Salmon

This is a great recipe for company. The end product is beautiful.

1/2 cup gluten free breadcrumbs
1/2 cup raw white hulled sesame seeds
1/2 teaspoon white pepper
1/2 teaspoon seafood seasoning
1 teaspoon salt
2 teaspoons smoked paprika

2 teaspoons chopped fresh parsley
1/4 cup plus 3 teaspoons dark (toasted) sesame oil
2 tablespoons avocado oil
2 pounds boneless, skinless salmon fillets, approx. 1 inch thick

Servings: 6

1. Mix together the breadcrumbs, sesame seeds, white pepper, salt, paprika, parsley, and 1/4 cup of the sesame oil.

2. Place a sauté pan over medium high heat and add the avocado oil.

3. Rub about 1 teaspoon of sesame oil on the top of each fillet, making sure it is well covered. Press fillets into the bread crumb mixture to coat well.

4. Place the breaded salmon, crumb side down, in the hot pan and sear for about 5 minutes or until evenly browned.

5. Turn the fillet over and finish cooking on the other side for about 5 minutes more.

Herb-Baked Salmon

1 lb. salmon
1/2 teaspoon salt
1/4 lemon squeezed
1/2 tablespoon Dijon mustard
1 tablespoon basil minced

1/4 teaspoon oregano minced
1/4 teaspoon thyme minced
1/4 teaspoon marjoram minced
2 cloves garlic, minced

Servings: 2-3

1. Preheat oven to 400° F.
2. Mince herbs and put in a small bowl with salt, mustard, lemon juice and garlic, stirring together to form a paste.
3. Put salmon on a piece of tin foil and curl up the sides. Place on a baking dish.
4. Slather salmon with herb/garlic paste.
5. Bake in oven for 10-15 min. or until salmon is cooked to your liking.

Grilled Salmon with Mango Salsa

Simple grilled salmon is always delicious. Serving it with Mango Salsa takes it to a whole new level.

2 6 oz. Salmon Fillets, wild caught
Olive Oil
Sea Salt and Pepper

For the Salsa

1 large ripe yet firm mango, diced into small pieces
1 medium red bell pepper, diced into small pieces
1 medium Jalapeno, seeded and diced into small pieces (if you can take the heat, add the seeds to the salsa)

1/4 cup red onion, diced finely
1 -2 tablespoons lemon/lime juice (+/- depending on your taste)
Salt to taste
1/4 cup of cilantro, chopped

Servings: 2

Salsa:

Combine the mango, red bell pepper, jalapeno pepper, red onion, lemon/lime juice, salt, and cilantro.

Salmon:

1. Preheat the grill. Drizzle olive oil on both sides of the salmon. If you don't like the skin on the fish, place the fish skin side down on the grill and grill for 3 min.

2. Flip the salmon. Easily remove the skin with tongs and grill for an additional 3-5 minutes (depending on thickness and doneness preference).

3. Flip again to finish 1-3 minutes (thickness/doneness)

4. Serve the salmon with the salsa on the side.

Shepherd's Pie

A fabulous dish for a winter's eve. Finding yams is worth the effort. They are less sweet than sweet potatoes.

1/4 cup dried currants
1 to 2 tablespoon avocado oil
1 pound ground lamb
1/2 teaspoon ground cinnamon
1/2 teaspoon ground ginger
1/4 teaspoon ground allspice
1/4 teaspoon ground cayenne pepper
Sea salt and freshly ground pepper to taste
1 large yellow onion, chopped
1 red bell pepper, chopped
2 to 4 carrots, scrubbed and chopped
1 jalapeno pepper, diced

6 cloves garlic, finely chopped
2 tablespoons tomato paste
1 cup red wine
1 (15-ounce can) chopped tomatoes with juice
1/4 cup chopped fresh flat leaf parsley, plus more for garnish
2 tablespoons chopped fresh oregano or 2 teaspoons dried
1 to 2 large yams or sweet potatoes, scrubbed and cut into 2" pieces
2 tablespoons coconut oil
1/4 cup chicken broth

1. Soak the currants in warm water for 30 minutes. Drain.

2. Heat 1 tablespoon of the avocado oil in a 6-quart saucepan over high heat. Add the lamb, cinnamon, ginger, allspice, cayenne, and salt and pepper and cook, stirring to break up the meat, until browned, about 5 minutes.

3. Transfer the lamb with a slotted spoon to a large strainer set over a bowl and drain; discard any liquid left in the pan. Return the pan to the heat. There should be about 1 tablespoon of fat remaining in the pan. If not, add another tablespoon of avocado oil and heat until it begins to shimmer.

4. Add the onions, bell pepper and carrot and cook until soft, about 5 minutes. Add the jalapeno and garlic and cook for 1 minute. Add the tomato paste and cook for 1 minute.

5. Return the lamb to the pan, add the wine, and cook, stirring occasionally, until almost completely evaporated, about 5 minutes. Add the tomato puree and currants and bring to a boil. Reduce the heat to medium-low and simmer until thickened, about 30 minutes. Stir in the parsley and oregano and season with salt and pepper.

6. Preheat the oven to 400° F.

7. Cover the cut-up yam with water in a saucepan with about ½ teaspoon salt and bring to a boil. Simmer for about 25 minutes or until soft. Drain the potatoes and mash by hand. Add the coconut oil and broth.

8. Cover the lamb mixture with the mashed yams starting around the edges to create a seal to prevent the mixture from bubbling up and smooth with a rubber spatula. Or, just spoon a mound of the yams around the top of the lamb dish. Put in the oven for 25 minutes. Let it rest for 10 minutes and then serve with parsley as a garnish.

Shrimp and Eggplant

1 eggplant
1 tablespoon avocado oil
2 tablespoons extra virgin olive oil
1 pound peeled raw shrimp
1 red bell pepper, diced
1 tablespoon fresh ginger, minced
1 tablespoon fresh garlic, minced
1/2 cup green onions, chopped

1/4 cup fresh cilantro, finely chopped
1 teaspoon cumin
1/2 teaspoon coriander
2 tablespoons red curry paste
1 tablespoon fish sauce
1 large egg, lightly beaten
3 tablespoons olive oil

1. Preheat oven to 400° F.

2. Take the eggplant and cut it into 2 pieces lengthwise. Make a series of parallel cuts, taking care not to cut through the skin. Brush the eggplant (cut sides) with ½ tablespoon of avocado oil on each side.

3. Place the eggplants cut side down on a roasting pan and brush the skin with ½ tablespoon avocado oil and bake for 15 minutes. Turn over after the initial 15 minutes and cook again 15 to 20 minutes or until the flesh is tender. Remove from oven and reduce the heat to 350° F.

4. In a small skillet, heat the remaining olive oil over a medium heat. Add the ginger, the garlic, and the red pepper, and cook for two minutes. Add the green onions and the cilantro and cook for another 2 to 3 minutes. Transfer to a medium bowl.

5. Once the eggplant is cool enough, scoop out the pulp leaving the skin intact and chop the eggplant pulp.

6. In the bowl containing the red bell pepper mixture; add the chopped eggplant, the shrimp, the beaten egg, the fish sauce and the 2 tablespoons curry paste and stir.

7. Insert the mixture evenly in the eggplant shell and place back in the oven for about 30 min until the stuffing is firm.

8. Garnish with cilantro leaves and serve.

Stuffed Sweet Potatoes

2 medium sweet potatoes
1 pound organic, grass-fed beef
1/2 sweet onion, chopped
Sea salt to taste

2 garlic cloves, minced
1 teaspoon ground cumin
1/2 medium avocado, chopped
Fresh chopped chives or cilantro leaves

Servings: 4

1. Preheat oven to 400° F.

2. Wash the sweet potatoes well with a brush, then pat dry.

3. Place them on a baking sheet and bake for 45 minutes. Remove from oven and decrease temperature to 375° F.

4. Brown ground beef in a skillet over medium heat. Add onion and cook until translucent 4 to 5 minutes. Add the garlic and cumin. Sauté for an additional 30 seconds.

5. When the sweet potatoes are cool enough to touch, split in half lengthwise. Set each sweet potato face up on an oiled baking sheet.

6. Scoop the meat mixture on top of each sweet potato. Bake for 20 minutes.

7. Serve topped with chopped avocado and sprinkled with chive and cilantro.

Quick Cassoulet

1-2 pints cherry or grape tomatoes
4 fresh sweet or hot chicken sausages,
   gluten free
4 large garlic cloves, smashed
olive oil

Balsamic vinegar
a few sprigs of fresh thyme or rosemary
1 15 oz. can white kidney, navy or
   cannellini beans, rinsed and drained

Servings: 4

1. Adjust oven rack to lowest position and heat oven to 425°F.

2. Scatter the tomatoes over the bottom of a baking dish. Add the garlic, lay the sausages over the top, and drizzle it all with some balsamic vinegar and olive oil. Toss in a few sprigs of thyme and/or rosemary, and sprinkle with salt and pepper.

3. When the tomatoes have split and the sausages are golden, remove the dish from the oven and stir in the beans. Return to the oven for 20 minutes or so, until the beans are cooked through and the sausages are even more golden.

4. Serve hot, with brown rice on the side.

Salmon with Miso and Asparagus

A beautiful dish for company and works well during the week, as well. If you have mastered how to steam fish in parchment paper that is a beautiful presentation, but aluminum foil wraps are quick and easy.

Aluminum foil for 4 packets

2 bunches of diagonally sliced asparagus
2 tablespoons fresh minced garlic,
  divided
2 teaspoons sesame oil
1/2 teaspoon sea salt
1 tablespoon ginger, minced
1 bunch of scallions, sliced

1/4 cup rice wine or dry white wine
1 tablespoon white miso
1 teaspoon sugar
1 tablespoon lemon juice
1 tablespoon sesame seeds
4 (6-ounce) salmon fillets

Servings: 4

1. Preheat oven to 450° F.

2. Combine asparagus with 1 tablespoon minced garlic, sesame oil and salt.

3. Combine the rest of the garlic with ginger, scallions, miso, sugar, and lemon juice in a small bowl.

4. Place about ¼ of the asparagus on the foil and top with a salmon filet and spoon about ¼ of the sauce on the fish. Wrap up the package and close with the seam on top.

5. Bake for 20 minutes or until the fish flakes.

6. Open each packet and sprinkle with sesame seeds. Serve.

Crispy Baked Tofu

I didn't really like tofu until I found this idea of baking it to crispiness before adding it to a stir fry or flavoring with additional ingredients. This is a great base for a healthy delicious snack, Tofu Snacks, and goes well with stir-fried vegetables.

1 16-ounce block extra-firm tofu, organic
    and non GMO
1 tablespoon extra-virgin olive oil

1 tablespoon tamari
1 tablespoon cornstarch or arrowroot
    starch or tapioca flour

1. Preheat oven to 400° F. Line a rimmed baking sheet with parchment paper. This is an important step, so the tofu doesn't stick to the pan.

2. Prep the tofu: Drain it well and use your hands to press out some of the water. Slice the tofu lengthwise so you have 3 slabs. Stack the slabs and slice through lengthwise to make 4 columns. Then slice across to make 5 columns.

3. Stack paper towels in several layers or a kitchen towel and lay sliced tofu on the paper towels in one even layer. Cover the tofu with other layers of paper towels or another kitchen towel. Place some heavy objects like large tomato cans on top of a dinner plate or a cast iron pan on top of the paper towels and let them sit for at least 10 minutes or 30 if you have the time.

4. Mix the olive oil, tamari and starch in a large bowl. Add the tofu and toss.

5. Arrange on the baking sheet in an even layer and bake for 30 minutes until golden brown, tossing the tofu halfway through the process.

Stir Fried Veggies with Tofu

This recipe can take extra time, but it is worth it. Instead of adding the tofu uncooked to the stir fry, bake it in the oven using the recipe for Crispy Baked Tofu. You can do this step ahead of time or you can bake the tofu while you are preparing the veggies.

2 tablespoons extra-virgin olive oil
2 cloves minced garlic
1 tablespoon ginger root, minced
1 small onion, cut into wedges
1 small head broccoli, cut into florets

1/2 cup snow peas
3/4 cup thinly sliced carrots
2 tablespoons tamari
1/4 cup chicken broth
1 recipe of Crispy Baked Tofu

1. In a wok or large skillet, heat the oil over medium heat. Stir fry the onions, garlic and ginger for about 5 minutes. Add the rest of the vegetables and stir fry for several minutes.

2. Add the tamari and chicken broth. Cook vegetables until tender but crisp.

3. Add the Crispy Baked Tofu. Enjoy!

Chocolate Chili

Simply a chili recipe with chocolate or cacao powder added. The added chocolate makes the turkey chili richer.

2 pounds ground turkey
2 onions, chopped
1 tablespoon plus 2 teaspoons chili powder
1 tablespoon ground cumin
2 to 4 tablespoons unsweetened cocoa powder
3 cloves garlic, minced
2 jalapeno peppers, seeded and minced

Two 15-ounce cans kidney beans, drained and rinsed
1 teaspoon cayenne pepper
1 teaspoon dried oregano
Two 15-ounce cans black beans, drained and rinsed
One 18-ounce can diced tomatoes
2 tablespoons tomato paste

Garnish if desired

Servings: 8

1. In a large Dutch oven over medium-high heat, add the ground turkey and cook for 2 minutes.

2. Add the onions, chili powder and cumin, and stir together. Add the cocoa, garlic and jalapenos, mix together and cook for 2 minutes.

3. Add kidney beans, cayenne pepper and oregano, and cook for another minute. Add the black beans, diced tomatoes, tomato paste, cover and simmer for 1 hour, stirring occasionally.

Garnish with sour cream, avocado, shredded cheese and/or chives if desired.

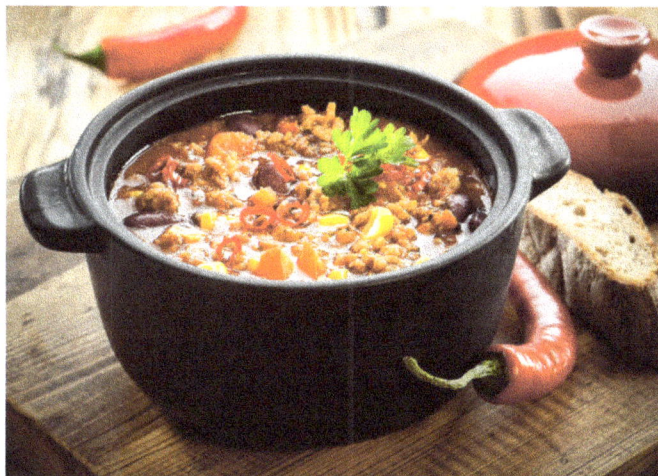

Beef with Bok Choy and Mushrooms

Flank steak is a nice lean cut of meat, but you need to be careful how you cook it and how you carve it to keep it tender.

1 tablespoon Dijon mustard
2 tablespoons fresh rosemary, stemmed
1 tablespoon minced fresh ginger
4 cloves garlic, minced
2 tablespoons freshly squeezed lemon
    juice
2 tablespoons red wine vinegar
4 tablespoons olive oil
1/2 teaspoons salt

1/2 teaspoon freshly ground black
    pepper
1½ pounds grass fed flank steak
6 to 8 scallions, sliced
1 head of Bok choy
8 oz. shitake mushrooms, sliced
1/2 cup chicken stock
1 tablespoon low sodium tamari sauce

Servings: 4

1. Mix the mustard, rosemary, ginger, garlic, lemon juice, vinegar, 3 tablespoons of oil and black pepper. Marinate the meat for at least 30 minutes.

2. Season the meat with salt. Heat a cast iron pan on high for a few minutes until it is hot. Lower the heat to medium high and sear the steak to desired doneness. For medium rare cook about 3 minutes per side. Remove the steak from the pan and allow it to rest for a few minutes. Slice the steak across the grain. This step is important to tenderize the steak. Look for the striations in the meat and cut crosswise. Set the pan aside.

3. In a separate pan, heat the oil over medium heat and sauté the onions for a few minutes. Add the Bok choy and the mushrooms and stir fry for a few minutes.

4. In the pan you used to cook the meat, add the stock and tamari, scraping up any bits on the bottom of the pan. Reduce the liquid to about one-half.

5. Place the veggies on a plate, put the steak on top and finish with the sauce in the pan.

Shish Kabobs – Chicken/Beef

I love shish kabobs in the summertime. All you need to do is marinate the protein, cut up some veggies and string them on grilling sticks.

Chicken Kabobs

For Greek Lemon Marinade

2 tablespoons extra virgin olive oil
1 lemon, juiced
3 cloves garlic, minced
1 tablespoon fresh or 1 teaspoon dried oregano

2 tablespoons fresh or 2 teaspoons dried basil
1/2 teaspoon salt
Freshly ground pepper

For Skewers

1 pound boneless organic chicken breast, cut into 1-inch cubes
Variety of veggies: onion wedges, peppers, zucchini, cherry tomatoes, mushrooms

Beef Kabobs

For Balsamic Vinaigrette Marinade

1 tablespoon Dijon mustard
2 tablespoons fresh rosemary, stemmed
4 cloves garlic, minced
2 tablespoons freshly squeezed lemon juice

2 tablespoons balsamic vinegar
1/4 cup olive oil
1/2 teaspoon salt
1/2 teaspoon freshly ground black pepper

For Skewers

1 pound sirloin steak, grass fed, cut into 1-inch cubes
Variety of veggies: onions, peppers, zucchini, cherry tomatoes

Servings: Each makes 4

1. Whisk together the ingredients for the marinade. Toss the meat in the mixture until evenly coated. Cover and marinate in refrigerator for 2 hours.

2. Cut vegetables into bite-size pieces.

3. Thread veggies on one set of skewers and cubes of meat on another. Baste with the marinade.

4. Grill meat kabobs directly over heat source for about 10 to 15 minutes, turning 1/4 rotation every 2 to 3 minutes, or until the meat is cooked throughout. Veggies can be grilled for a shorter period of time.

Pan-Seared Scallops with Garlic and Paprika

Scallops are a bit expensive but a great treat. Garlic is a must in this recipe.

1 tablespoon olive oil
1 pound scallops
Sea salt and pepper

Paprika, preferably smoked
2-3 cloves of garlic, minced
1/3 cup white wine, water or clam broth

1. Warm a skillet over medium high heat. Add the olive oil.
2. Salt, pepper and add paprika to both sides of the scallops.
3. Sauté scallops in oil for about 3 minutes per side.
4. Remove from the pan.
5. Add the minced garlic and sauté for 30 seconds. Add broth or water and reduce by half.
6. Add the scallops back to the pan for 2 minutes and serve.

Baked Flounder

Olive oil to grease the pan
4 6- to 8-ounce flounder fillets
Salt and freshly cracked black pepper

1 lime, finely grated zest and juice
2 tablespoons butter, clarified

Servings: 4

1. Preheat oven to 375° F. Coat a large cast iron pan with a little olive oil.
2. Rinse fish and pat dry; place on the cast iron pan.
3. Season each fillet with salt, cracked pepper, lime zest and lime juice.
4. Add fish to the pan.
5. Pour about 1½ teaspoon clarified butter on each fillet and cook in the oven for 8 to 12 minutes.

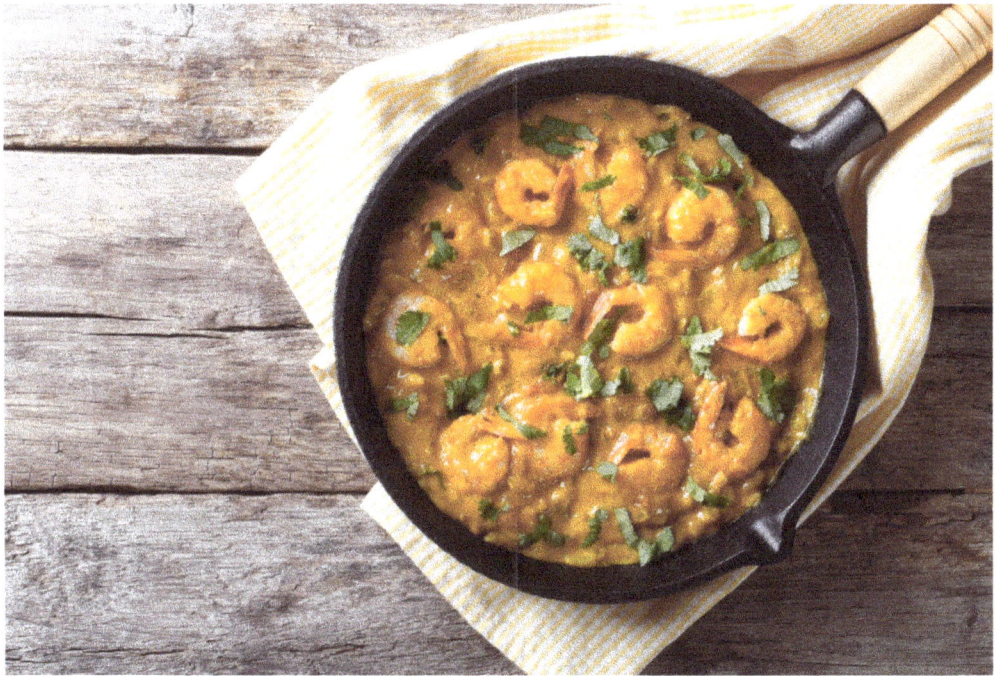

Above: Entrees – Shrimp Curry

Below: Entrees – Pan-Seared Scallops

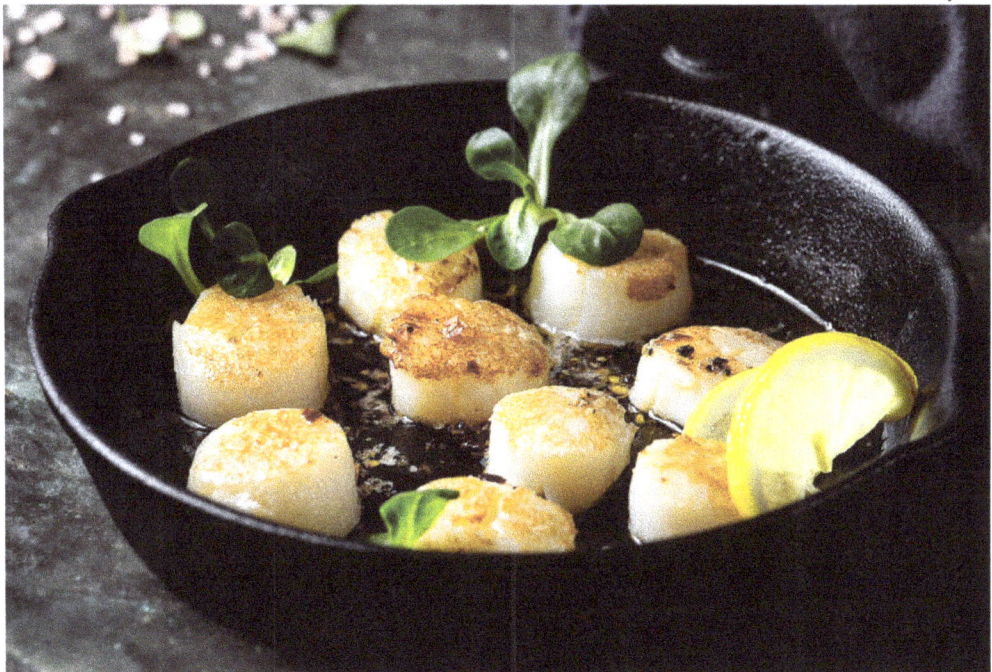

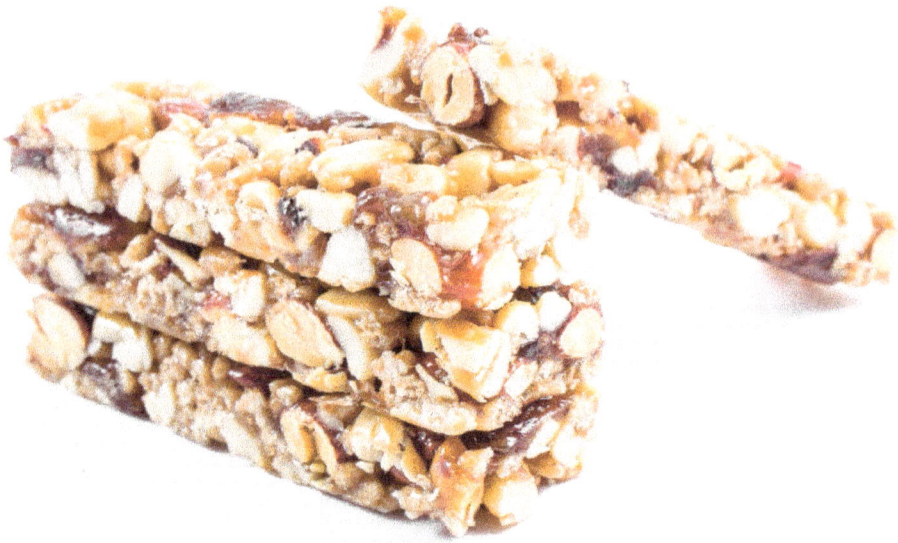

Above: Snacks – Grain–Free Granola Bars

Below: Snacks – Tofu Snacks

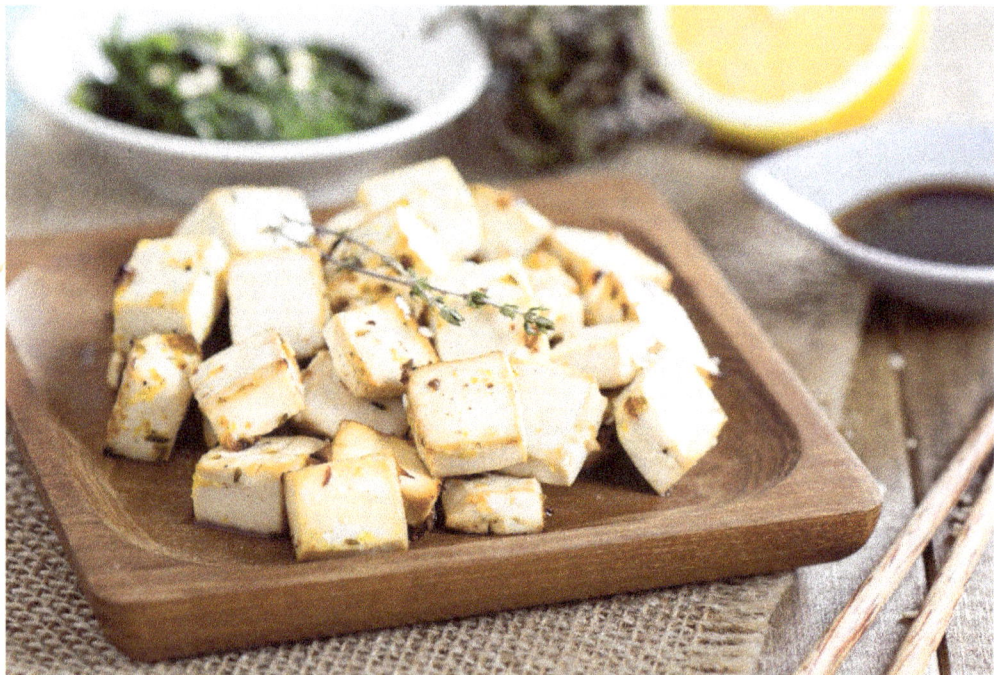

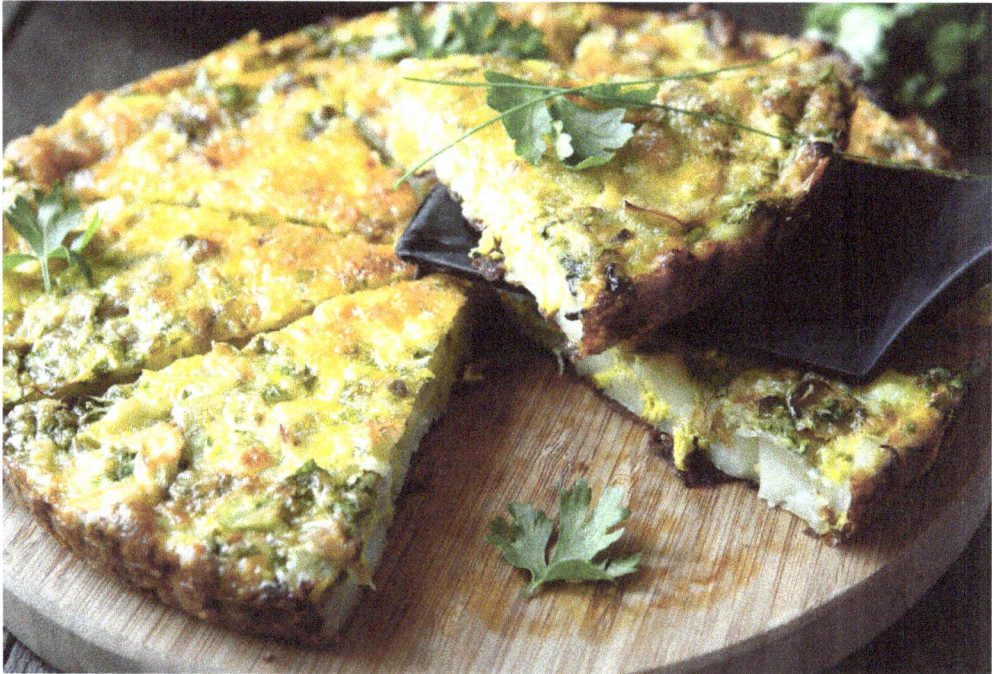

Above: Breakfasts – Frittata

Below: Breakfasts – Chia Seed Pudding

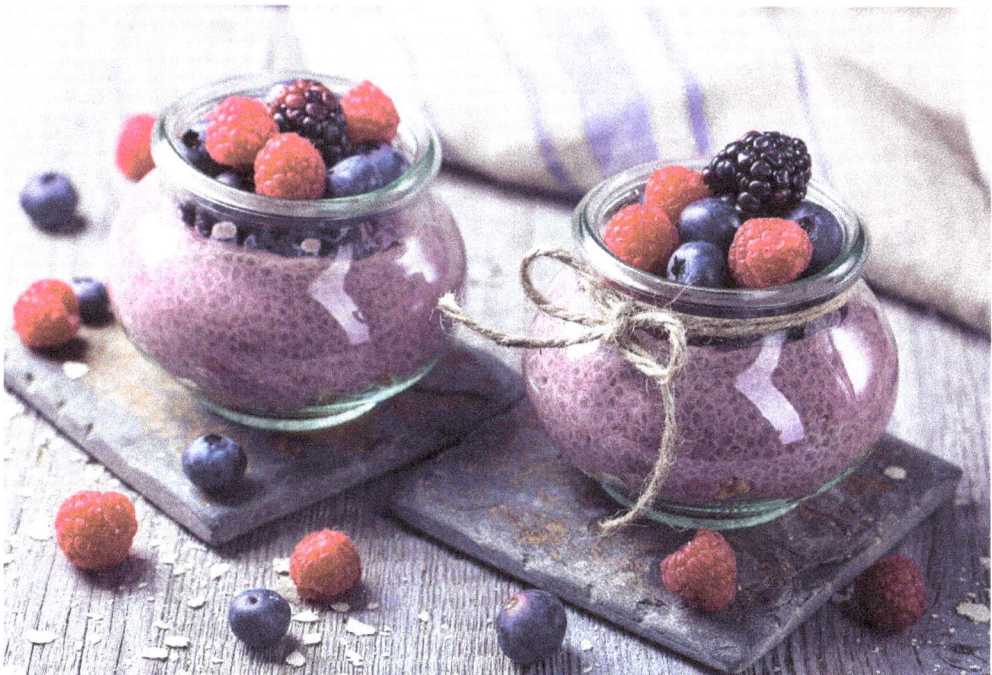

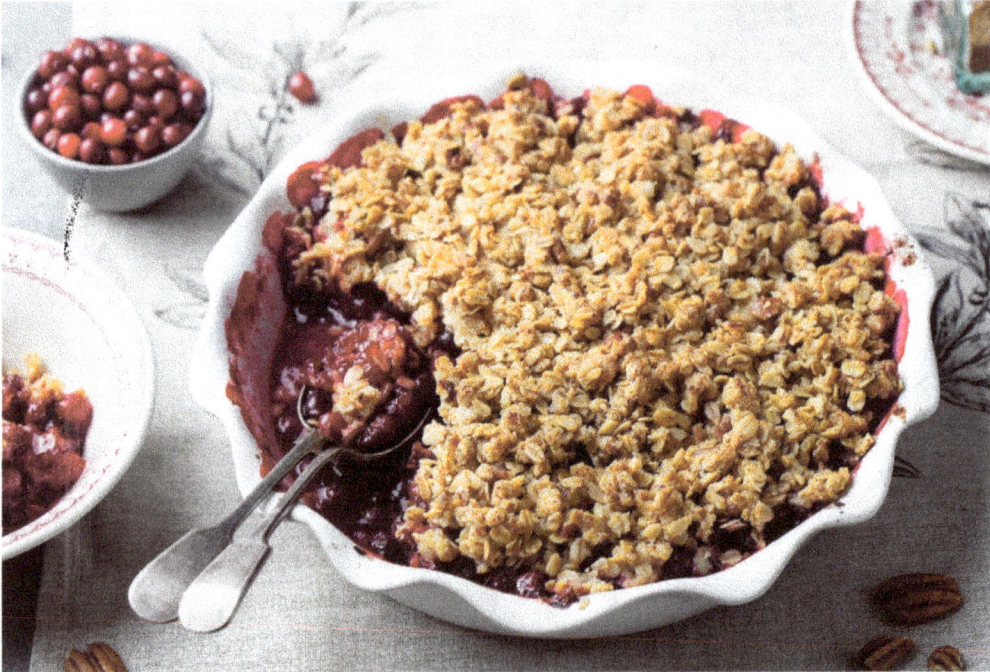

Above: Desserts – Cranberry-Apple

Below: Desserts – Chocolate Dipped Banana Bites

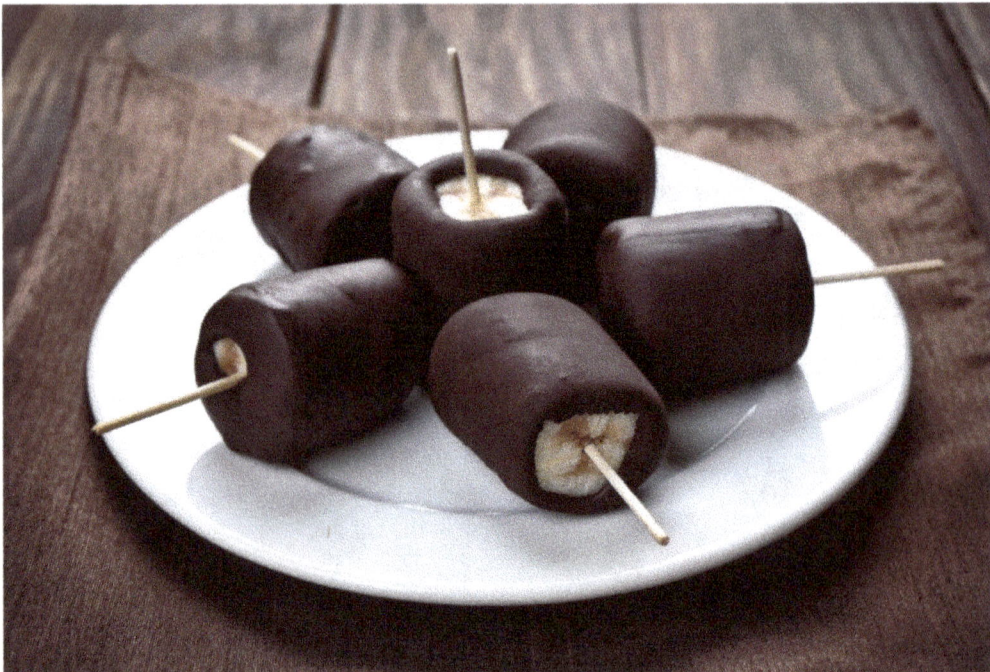

Pan-Seared Flounder and Green Beans

A simple, easy but delicious treatment of flounder. Make sure you don't overcook it.

2 teaspoons chopped fresh oregano or 1 teaspoon dried, plus more for garnish
2 tablespoons chopped fresh or 2 teaspoons dried parsley
1/4 cup brown rice flour
Sea salt and freshly ground pepper
4 6-ounce flounder fillets

4 tablespoons unsalted butter, clarified*
1/2 pound thin green beans or haricots verts
1 clove garlic, chopped
1 cup grape or cherry tomatoes, halved
2 tablespoons fresh lemon juice
Lemon wedges for garnish

Servings: 4

1. Combine the flour, oregano and parsley in a shallow dish. Season with salt and pepper.

2. Place a large skillet over medium-high heat. Dredge the fish in the flour mixture, shaking off the excess. Melt 3 tablespoons butter in the skillet, then add 2 fillets and cook until golden brown on the bottom, about 4 minutes. Flip and cook through, 1 to 2 more minutes. Transfer to a plate and keep warm. Repeat with the remaining 2 fillets.

3. Add the green beans and garlic to the skillet and cook about 2 minutes. Season with salt and pepper, then add the tomatoes and cook until just softened, about 1 more minute. Stir in the lemon juice and 1/4 cup water, then cover and cook until the beans are tender, about 3 more minutes. Remove from the heat and stir in the remaining 1 tablespoon butter until just melted.

4. Divide the fish and vegetables among plates. Garnish with lemon wedges and oregano. This makes 4 portions so serve 2 and save 2 for another meal.

*clarified butter—Melt a stick of butter and pour off the clarified butter leaving the white diary solids in the pan. Store and use for additional recipes.

Codfish with Capers, Lemon and Thyme

2 6 oz. fillets of cod
1/4 cup capers
Grated zest of one lemon
1/2 teaspoon of thyme
1 tablespoon extra-virgin olive oil

Sea salt
Fresh ground pepper to taste
4 cups of Swish chard, washed and
    roughly chopped

Servings: 2

1. Heat oven to 400° F.

2. In a baking dish place the codfish, grated lemon zest, capers and thyme.

3. Drizzle olive oil over the top. Season with salt and pepper.

4. Cover with foil. Bake for 10 to 15 min, depends on the fish. When it flakes easily with a fork it's done.

5. Meanwhile, heat a sauté pan and add 1 tablespoon oil. When hot, add the Swiss chard; cover and let steam for 2 minutes.

6. Serve the fish on a bed of chard. Spoon juices and capers over the fish. Garnish with thyme.

You can substitute a local white fish, red snapper or haddock.

Baked Cod with Avocado Salsa

1 pound of codfish
1 avocado, mashed
1 tomato, chopped
1/2 cup red onion, chopped
1/4 cup capers, drained

1/4 cup fresh cilantro
1/2 teaspoon cumin
pinch of cayenne
2 tablespoon lime juice

Servings: 2

1. Heat oven to 400° F.

2. Place the cod in a baking dish and drizzle with olive oil. Season with salt and pepper. Cover with foil and bake for 10 to 15 min depending on thickness of fish. When it flakes easily with a fork, it's done.

3. While the fish is cooking combine the rest of the ingredients. Serve the avocado salsa over the fish.

Marinated Shrimp Kabobs

A great dish for company. You can reduce the portion for appetizers or increase for a main dish.

1 lb. raw shrimp, large or jumbo
1/4 cup olive oil
1/4 cup lemon juice
3 large garlic cloves (minced finely)
1 teaspoon sea salt
1/2 teaspoon pepper

1 tablespoon chopped parsley, plus 1/4
   cup for garnish*
2 teaspoons hot sauce
1 tablespoon brown sugar
1 teaspoon smoked paprika

Servings: 2-3

1. Add all ingredients to a large bowl and stir to combine.

2. Refrigerate for 30 minutes. Don't overdo it because the shrimp will get tough.

3. If you are using wood skewers, soak them in cold water while the shrimp marinates.

4. Grill for about 2 to 3 minutes per side.

5. Garnish with extra parsley.

*You can add other herbs like thyme, rosemary or dill to amplify the flavor.

Mushroom Steaks with Kale and Red Onion

4 Portabella mushrooms, stems removed
1 bunch of kale, stems removed, leaves
   torn into smaller pieces
1 medium sized red onion, cut into ½"
   thick rounds

2 tablespoons olive oil
Sea salt, to taste
Freshly cracked black pepper

For the Marinade
½ cup extra-virgin olive oil
4 tablespoons lemon juice
2 tablespoons wheat-free tamari

1 teaspoon chopped fresh rosemary
1 teaspoon fresh thyme
2 garlic cloves, roughly chopped

Servings: 2

1. Preheat oven to 400° F. Whisk together marinade ingredients and coat the mushrooms gently. Let stand at room temperature for 30 minutes

2. Toss the kale in a bowl with the red onions. Drizzle with olive oil, sea salt and black pepper.

3. Spread the mushrooms on one half of a baking sheet and the kale red onion mixture on the other half. Drizzle with pan juices.

4. Bake for 10 minutes until the mushrooms are tender and the kale is wilted.

Sweet Potato Chili

A great dinner recipe following a day of snowshoeing or other exercise. It is a heavy dish and a little goes a long way. Serve with a green salad.

2 tablespoons olive oil
1 onion, chopped
3 garlic cloves, minced
2 carrots, diced
3 celery stalks, diced
8 ounces mushrooms, sliced
2 sweet potatoes, peeled and diced
2 parsnips, peeled and diced
1 pound ground beef, grass fed
1 pound ground chicken sausage, gluten-free
28 ounces of peeled tomatoes
2 tablespoons tomato paste

1 tablespoon chili powder (more or less depending upon your taste preferences)
1 teaspoon ground cumin
1/4 teaspoon cayenne pepper
1 teaspoon dried oregano
2 bay leaves
2 teaspoons smoked paprika
1 teaspoon salt
1/4 cup cilantro
1/4 teaspoon (approximately) freshly ground pepper

Servings: 8

1. In a large Dutch oven, brown hamburger and sausage. Once browned, remove, drain and set aside.

2. Add in olive oil to the Dutch oven over low-medium heat. Once hot, add chopped onion, celery, garlic cloves, mushrooms, sweet potatoes and parsnips. Cook until onion is translucent.

3. Add in spices, mixing to combine.

4. Add tomatoes, tomato paste and ground beef and sausage.

5. Simmer until veggies are tender.

6. Season with additional salt and pepper, if needed.

7. Serve and garnish with cilantro.

Chicken in a Pot

1 chicken, about 3 pounds, cut into
  serving pieces
1 teaspoon freshly ground black pepper
3 tablespoons fresh thyme leaves or 3
  teaspoons dried
1 teaspoon chopped fresh rosemary
1 tablespoon extra-virgin olive oil

1 1/2 teaspoons unsalted butter,
  clarified*
1/2 cup minced yellow onion
2 cloves garlic, minced
4 cups chopped canned tomatoes and
  their juice
16 oil-cured black olives (optional)

1. Rub the chicken pieces all over with the pepper, half of the thyme and half of the rosemary. In a Dutch oven large enough to eventually hold all the chicken pieces, heat the olive oil and butter over medium-high heat. When it is nearly smoking, add the chicken pieces a few at a time. Reduce the heat to medium, and sauté for 2 to 3 minutes until lightly browned.

2. Turn the pieces over and cook for another 1 to 2 minutes to brown the other side. Remove to a bowl when done and repeat with the remaining chicken pieces. Add the onion and garlic and continue to cook for another 1 to 2 minutes.

3. Pour in the chopped tomatoes and their juices, scraping up any bits clinging to the pot. Return the chicken and any collected juices to the pot, spooning the sauce over the chicken. Cover, reduce the heat to medium-low, and cook until the juices run clear when the thickest part of a thigh is pierced with a knife, 75 to 90 minutes.

4. Remove the cover, increase the heat to medium, add the olives, and cook for another 5 minutes or so, or as needed to reduce and thicken the sauce. Stir in the remaining thyme and rosemary and serve hot.

*To clarify butter, melt a stick of butter over medium-high heat until the mixture bubbles. Scrape the bubbles off and pour the golden liquid that remains into a bowl, leaving the white milk solids behind. Your butter is now dairy free.

Pork Tenderloin with Chicken Sausage and Black Beans

A hearty dish for midwinter. The dish is calorie dense so watch your portion and keep the rest of the meal light.

2 tablespoons olive oil, cold-pressed
1 pound gluten free chicken sausage
1½ pounds pork tenderloin, cut into 1½ inch cubes
1 onion, chopped
1/2 red pepper, chopped
3 cloves garlic, minced
1 cup canned crushed tomatoes

1/4 cup cilantro, chopped plus more for garnish
1 bay leaf
1½ cups chicken stock, canned and low sodium
1/2 teaspoon salt
3 15-ounce cans of black beans, drained and rinsed
1/8 teaspoon fresh ground black pepper

Servings: 8

1. In a large pot, heat ½ tablespoon of oil over moderate heat. Add the sausage and cook, turning until browned, about 8 minutes.

2. Add 1 tablespoon oil to the pot and raise the heat to moderately high. Add about half of the pork to the pan and cook until the meat begins to brown, about 3 minutes. Remove. Repeat with the remaining pork. Remove.

3. Add the remaining ½ tablespoon oil to the pot and reduce the heat to moderately low. Add the onion and red pepper and cook, stirring occasionally, until onions are translucent, about 5 to 10 minutes. Add the garlic and cook stirring, for 30 seconds. Add the tomatoes, cilantro and bay leaf. Cook, stirring frequently, for 5 minutes.

4. Add the sausage, the pork tenderloin with any accumulated juices, the stock and the salt. Bring to a boil, reduce the heat and simmer, partially covered for 15 minutes. Remove the bay leaf.

5. Meanwhile, puree 1 cup of beans and a little of the liquid from the simmering stew in a food processor or blender. Stir the pureed and whole beans and the pepper into the stew and continue cooking for 5 minutes. Serve with cilantro sprinkled on top.

Roasted Pork Tenderloin with Fennel and Garlic

Pork tenderloin is a lean cut of meat that is easy to use, fast cooking and goes with a lot of flavors.

12 garlic cloves, peeled
3 pounds fennel bulbs (3 to 4), fronds
    and stalks removed, bulbs cored and
    cut into eighths lengthwise
3 tablespoons olive oil

Coarse salt and ground pepper
2 pork tenderloins (about 1 pound each)
1/2 teaspoon dried oregano
1/2 teaspoon garlic powder

Servings: 4

1. Preheat oven to 475° F. On a large rimmed baking sheet, toss garlic, fennel and 2 tablespoons oil; season with salt and pepper. Roast 10 minutes.

2. Rub pork with remaining tablespoon oil; season with oregano, garlic powder, salt and pepper.

3. Remove baking sheet from oven, and push fennel and garlic to sides of sheet.

4. Place pork in center, and roast 20 to 25 minutes, until an instant-read thermometer inserted in thickest part registers 145.

5. Transfer pork to a cutting board and let rest at least 5 minutes before thinly slicing. Serve pork with fennel and garlic.

Pork Tenderloin with Roasted Apples and Onions

A great autumn dish for the peak of the apple season.

1/4 cup balsamic vinegar
2 tablespoons maple syrup
1/2 teaspoon dried thyme
1/2 teaspoon dried rosemary
3 medium red apples, halved and cored,
   each cut into 8 wedges

1 large red onion, halved and sliced into
   1/2-inch-thick pieces
1 tablespoon olive oil
Coarse salt and ground pepper
2 pork tenderloins (12 ounces each),
   trimmed of excess fat

Servings: 4

1. Place one oven rack in top third of oven, and another rack in bottom third. Preheat oven to 450° F.

2. Make glaze: In a small saucepan, bring herbs, vinegar and maple syrup to a boil over high heat; cook, stirring occasionally, until mixture has reduced to 1/4 cup, 3 to 4 minutes. Remove from heat; transfer 1 tablespoon to a small bowl for drizzling and set aside. Reserve the rest of the glaze in saucepan.

3. On a large rimmed baking sheet, toss apples and onion with oil. Season with salt and pepper; arrange in a single layer, and roast until golden, about 15 minutes. Remove from oven and toss.

4. Meanwhile, line another rimmed baking sheet with aluminum foil; place pork on foil. Season generously with salt and pepper and brush with glaze from saucepan.

5. Return apples and onion to oven, on bottom rack. Place pork on top rack; roast 10 minutes. Remove pork from oven and brush with glaze (discard any remaining in pan). Roast until pork registers 145° F on an instant-read thermometer, and apples and onion are tender, about 10 minutes more.

6. Transfer pork to a cutting board and let rest 10 minutes. Slice 1/4 inch thick. Drizzle with reserved tablespoon glaze. Serve with apples, and onion.

Pork Tenderloin with Italian Herb Seasoned Rub

Very flavorful and a snap to make. Pork tenderloin is great because you can have it on the table in about 30 minutes or less.

1 teaspoon garlic powder
1 teaspoon Italian herbs
1 teaspoon ground cumin
1 teaspoon ground coriander
1 teaspoon dried thyme
1 teaspoon smoked paprika

1 teaspoon fennel seeds, ground
1/4 teaspoon cayenne pepper
3/4 teaspoon salt
1¼ pounds pork tenderloin
1 tablespoon olive oil
1 teaspoon minced garlic

Servings: 2

1. Preheat the oven to 450° F.

2. In separate bowl mix dry ingredients: garlic powder, Italian herbs, cumin, coriander, thyme, fennel, cayenne pepper and salt. Sprinkle the rub over the tenderloin with a dry hand, then rub the pork with the seasoning over both sides of the meat, pressing gently so the seasoning adheres well to the tenderloin.

3. In a large skillet over medium-high heat, add the olive oil and heat. Add the minced garlic and sauté, stirring, for 1 minute. Put tenderloin in the pan searing each side for about 2 minutes, using tongs to turn the meat. Transfer meat to a roasting pan and bake for 20 minutes or until instant read thermometer reads 145° F.

4. Let the tenderloin rest for 5 minutes. Slice and serve.

Quick Peanut Quinoa Casserole

1 cup quinoa
2 cups water
1/2 cup chopped red onion

1/2 cup chopped red pepper
1/4 cup chopped fresh cilantro
2 cups chopped spinach or Swiss chard

Peanut Sauce:

1/4 cup peanut butter
2 tablespoons rice vinegar
1 tablespoon tamari, low sodium
4 cloves garlic chopped

1 teaspoon ginger grated
1/2 teaspoon hot red pepper flakes
4 tablespoons water

Optional Garnish:

Chopped fresh herbs (basil, cilantro, mint)
Roasted peanuts (shelled)
Lime wedges
Crushed red pepper

1. Bring 2 cups of water to a boil in a medium saucepan. Add quinoa and simmer briskly until quinoa is tender, about 15 minutes.

2. In the meantime, whisk together peanut butter, rice vinegar, tamari, garlic, ginger, red pepper flakes and water until the sauce is pourable.

3. Stir in cooked quinoa, onion, red pepper, cilantro and spinach.

4. Serve with fresh herbs, peanuts, lime wedges, and crushed red pepper, if using.

5. Serve warm or at room temperature.

BREAKFASTS

One of the most important ways to start the day. When you eat breakfast is up to you. Make sure it works for you. If you have been struggling with your weight, you may try eating later in the morning when you feel you need it instead of eating first thing because you think you "should." Just make sure you have a plan.

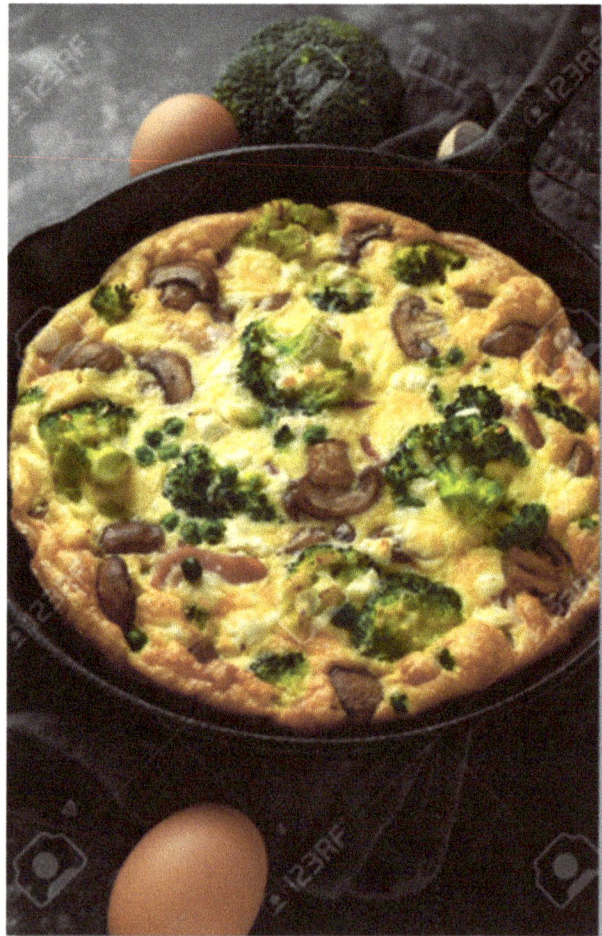

Autumn Breakfast Casserole

I love to make breakfast casseroles for those times that I have overnight guests. Make them the evening before and refrigerate overnight. No mess or fuss in the morning. Serve it with a fruit salad.

1 tablespoon olive oil
12 eggs
2 cups winter squash cubed (butternut or delicata)
2 cups greens (kale, chard, and/or spinach)

1 cup Brussels sprouts, shaved
1 cup mushrooms, sliced
1 leek, diced
2 links of chicken sausage, sliced
1 tablespoon fresh thyme - chopped
1/4 teaspoon each: salt & pepper

Servings: 10 - 12

1. Preheat oven to 375° F. Grease a 9x13" pan with the oil.

2. Crack eggs in a large mixing bowl and whisk until creamy.

3. Prepare the rest of the ingredients and add to the eggs. Mix thoroughly and pour into greased pan.

4. Place in the oven and bake for 40 minutes, or until the egg mixture is cooked through.

5. Remove and let cool for a few minutes, and serve, or let cool completely and store in fridge to reheat and serve for breakfast throughout the week.

Tofu Scramble

1 tablespoon olive oil
1/2 cup onion, chopped
1 16-ounce block firm tofu, organic and non-GMO
2 tablespoons nutritional yeast
1/2 to 1 teaspoon salt, to taste

1/4 teaspoon turmeric
1/4 teaspoon garlic powder
1 cup packed baby spinach leaves
2 tablespoons plant milk (almond, coconut, oat, cashew), unsweetened and unflavored

1. Heat the olive oil in a pan over medium heat. Add onion and sauté for 3 to 5 minutes. Add tofu to the pan and mash with a potato masher or a fork. (You can also crumble it into the pan with your hands).

2. Cook, stirring frequently, for 3-4 minutes until the water from the tofu is mostly gone.

3. Add the nutritional yeast, salt, turmeric and garlic powder. Cook and stir constantly for about 5 minutes.

4. Pour the plant milk into the pan and stir to mix. Serve immediately with sliced avocado and tomatoes.

Spring Vegetable Egg Casserole

This is an easy egg casserole. Serve for breakfast, brunch, or even dinner!

1 tablespoon olive oil
1/2 cup diced yellow onion
2 cups asparagus, cut into 1-inch pieces
6 cups packed fresh spinach leaves
2 cloves garlic, minced
2 tablespoons freshly chopped dill

2 green onions, sliced
2 tablespoons nutritional yeast flakes
12 large eggs, whisked
1/2 cup Almond Breeze Original Almond
  Milk
Salt and black pepper, to taste

Servings: 10-12

1. Preheat oven to 350° F. Spray or brush a 9×13 inch baking dish with olive oil.

2. In a large skillet, heat olive oil over high heat. Add the onion and cook until tender, about 3 minutes. Stir in the asparagus, spinach, and garlic. Cook for 4 minutes, or until vegetables are tender and spinach is wilted. Stir in the dill, half of the green onions and nutritional yeast flakes. Season with salt and black pepper, to taste. Pour vegetable mixture into prepared pan and spread out evenly.

3. In a medium bowl, combine eggs and milk. Whisk well. Season with salt and black pepper, to taste. Pour egg mixture evenly over the veggies.

4. Bake for 30-35 minutes or until eggs are set and slightly golden around the edges. A knife inserted into the center should come out clean. Remove from oven and let cool for 10 minutes. Garnish if desired. Cut into squares and serve warm.

Note-this casserole reheats well and can be made a day in advance.

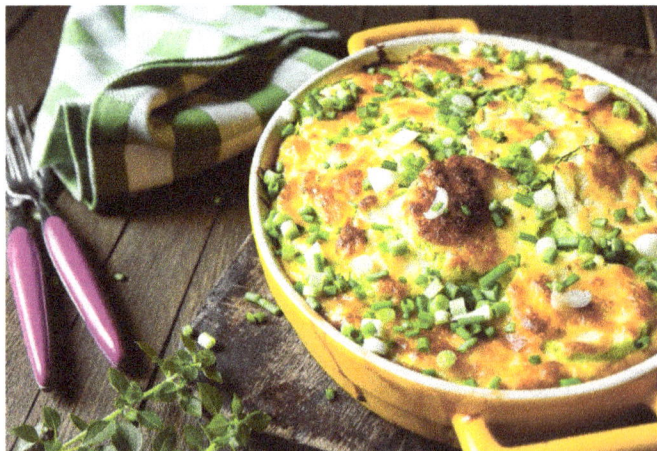

Broccoli & Zucchini Frittata

Frittatas are easy to make and great for a last-minute dinner.

1 small head broccoli, cut into bite-sized
  pieces
1 small zucchini, cut into bite-sized pieces
2 small leeks, sliced
2 tablespoons extra-virgin olive oil

1 teaspoon dried or 1 tablespoon fresh
  basil
8 eggs
1/4 cup water
1/2 teaspoon salt
1/4 teaspoon pepper

1. Preheat broiler. Make sure the top oven rack is positioned about 4 inches from the broiler unit.

2. Over medium heat in a large sauté* pan sauté broccoli, zucchini and leeks until crisp tender, about 6-7 minutes in oil. Reduce heat to low.

3. Whisk eggs and water in a bowl until well blended. Add salt, pepper and basil.

4. Spread veggies in the pan so they are evenly distributed. Pour egg mixture over veggies. Cover and cook for 2 minutes. Remove cover, place sauté pan in oven and broil for 3 to 4 minutes. To test press the center of the frittata lightly with your finger. When it is firm, it is done.

*Make sure the handle of your saute pan is heat tolerant

Sunnyside Veggie Eggs with Avocado

2 teaspoons extra-virgin olive oil
1/2 cup onion, chopped
Salt and pepper to taste
1/2 cup mushrooms, sliced

1 cup Swiss chard, packed
2 pasture raised eggs
1/4 to 1/2 avocado, sliced

1. In a small pan heat olive oil over medium heat. Add the onions and sauté for 2 to 3 minutes. Add the mushroom and Swiss chard and sauté for another 2 to 3 minutes.

2. Push the veggies to the side of the pan to make room for the eggs. Add a bit more oil if needed. Cover the pan for about 4 to 5 minutes depending on how you like your eggs.

3. Slide the contents of the pan on to a plate. Serve with a healthy serving of avocado.

Kale, Red Onion and Mushroom Frittata

1 bunch Tuscan kale, cut into bite-sized
   pieces
1/2 cup red onion, diced
8 ounces baby Bella mushrooms
2 tablespoons extra-virgin olive oil

1 teaspoon dried or 1 tablespoon fresh
   thyme
8 eggs
1/4 cup water
1/2 teaspoon salt
1/4 teaspoon pepper

1. Preheat broiler. Make sure the top oven rack is positioned about 4 inches from the broiler unit.

2. Over medium heat in a large sauté pan* sauté red onion in oil for 5 minutes. Add kale and mushrooms and sauté about 6-7 minutes in oil. Reduce heat to low.

3. Whisk eggs and water in a bowl until well blended. Add salt, pepper and thyme.

4. Spread veggies in the pan so they are evenly distributed. Pour egg mixture over veggies. Cover and cook for 2 minutes. Remove cover, place the sauté pan in the oven and broil for 3 to 4 minutes. To test press the center of the frittata lightly with your finger. If it is firm, it is done.

*Make sure the handle of your pan is heat tolerant.

Hormone Balancing Smoothies

You can pack a lot of nutrition and goodies in a smoothie. It is one of the best ways I have found to add herbs to my routine to help with hormonal imbalance.

Standard Recipe

1 scoop of protein powder, Innate Vegan Protein or Pure PaleoMeal*

1 cup of plant milk; almond, rice, coconut, hemp

3/4 cup frozen berries

Handful of greens; spinach, kale, swiss chard, dandelion

Handful of parsley or cilantro

1 tablespoon chia seeds or ground flax seeds

Blend in blender.

Smoothies for specific hormone challenges:

Cortisol—Make the standard recipe. Add ashwagandha powder.

Estrogen Dominance—Make the standard recipe. Increase the seeds for fiber to help you eliminate estrogen and make sure you use parsley and greens to support your liver. Dandelion is especially good.

Estrogen Deficiency—Make the standard recipe. Choose flax seeds for their phytoestrogen. Add gelatinized maca** in ¼ teaspoon increments up to 1 to 2 tablespoons to boost libido and endurance.

Thyroid—Make the standard recipe. Either choose swiss chard or spinach or lightly steam the kale. Add 1 to 2 Brazil nuts for selenium and ½ teaspoon dried seaweed for iodine. Avoid iodine if you have Hashimoto's.

*You can order these protein powders in my dispensary at www.supplements.smartnutritionllc.com. Just use your email to set up an account and create a password. You can also find a protein base which contains a non-whey protein, 0 sugar and at least 15 to 20 grams of protein. Good tasting dairy and gluten free protein powders are not easy to find so that is why I make this specific recommendation.

https://www.mountainroseherbs.com is a great place to purchase high quality herbs.

**Gelatinized maca is easier to absorb and is available in my dispensary (link above).

Smoothies Recipes

I find my clients can get tired of smoothies if they keep having the same berry smoothie day in and day out. Try some of these alternatives. I love the Pumpkin one especially as the days start to get cooler and shorter.

In each recipe add all ingredients and blend – on High where ice or frozen ingredients are used.

Detox Berry Smoothie
1 scoop of protein powder
1/2 cup frozen organic raspberries
1/2 cup frozen organic blueberries
1 cup plant milk, unsweetened

Cherry Zinger Smoothie
1 scoop of protein powder
3/4 cup frozen organic cherries
3/4 cup plant milk, unsweetened
Thumbnail size piece of ginger, washed and unpeeled

Strawberry "Chocolate" Smoothie
1 scoop protein powder
1 cup frozen organic strawberries
1 cup plant milk, unsweetened
1 to 2 tablespoons carob powder or natural unprocessed cocoa, unsweetened
Stevia to taste

Southern Style Smoothie
1 scoop of protein powder
1/2 cup fresh or frozen organic peaches
1/2 cup fresh or frozen blueberries
1 cup plant milk, unsweetened
Pinch of cinnamon

Peach Ginger Smoothie
1 scoop of protein powder
1 cup frozen sliced peaches
1 cup of almond milk, unsweetened
1 chunk of fresh ginger root
Add-ins to balance hormones

Spiced Pumpkin Smoothie
1 scoop of protein powder
1 can pureed pumpkin
1½ cups plant milk, unsweetened
3 or 4 ice cubes
1/2 teaspoon cinnamon
1/8 teaspoon nutmeg
1 teaspoon vanilla

Banana Ginger Smoothie
1 scoop protein powder
1/2 frozen banana
1 cup coconut milk, unsweetened
1 small chunk of fresh ginger root
1/4 teaspoon cinnamon

Strawberry Kiwi Smoothie
1 scoop of protein powder
1/2 banana, frozen
1 kiwi, peeled and sliced
5 frozen strawberries
1 cup plant milk, unsweetened

Chocolate Cherry Smoothie

1 scoop of protein powder
3/4 cup frozen dark cherries
3/4 cup plant milk, unsweetened
2 to 3 ice cubes
*2 tablespoon dark cocoa, natural and
    unsweetened*
Cacao nibs, for topping

Sprinkle top of smoothie with cacao nibs.

Pina Colada Smoothie

1 scoop protein powder
1/2 cup frozen pineapple chunks
1/4 frozen banana
1 cup coconut milk, unsweetened
1 tablespoon coconut oil
1/4 teaspoon coconut extract
*Unsweetened shredded coconut, for
    topping*

Sprinkle top of smoothie with unsweetened coconut.

Chai Banana Smoothie

1 scoop of protein powder
1/2 frozen banana
1 cup plant milk, unsweetened
*1/2 teaspoon chai spice mixture (see
    below)*
Cacao nibs, for topping
Sprinkle top of smoothie with cacao nibs.

> ### Chai spice mixture:
> *2 teaspoons cinnamon*
> *2 teaspoons cardamom*
> *1 teaspoon ginger*
> *1 teaspoon cloves*
> *1 teaspoon nutmeg*

Mix all ingredients in a small bowl. Store in air-tight container for up to 3 months.

Creamsicle Smoothie

1 scoop of protein powder
1/2 cup frozen mango
3 tablespoons orange juice concentrate
1 cup coconut milk, unsweetened
*Shredded unsweetened coconut, for
    topping*

Sprinkle top of smoothie with unsweetened coconut.

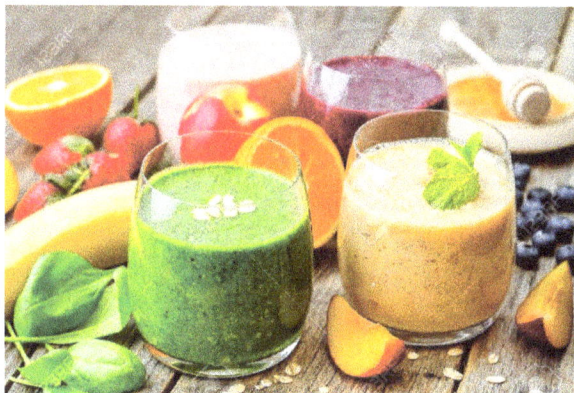

Quinoa Breakfast Skillet

4 slices thick-cut uncured bacon,
   chopped
1 tablespoon olive oil
1 small sweet potato, chopped
1/2 red onion, chopped
1/2 red pepper, chopped
1/2 green pepper, chopped

1 cup sliced mushrooms, chopped
2 garlic cloves, minced
1/2 cup uncooked quinoa, rinsed
1 cup low-sodium vegetable or chicken
   stock (or water)
4 eggs, cooked your desired way
Salt and pepper to taste

1. Heat a large skillet over medium heat and add bacon. Cook until fat is rendered and bacon is crispy, then remove bacon with a slotted spoon and place on a paper towel to drain.

2. Pour off bacon fat from pan and wipe with a paper towel, carefully.

3. Add oil to skillet. Reduce heat to medium-low and add sweet potato, onions, peppers, mushrooms and garlic to the skillet, tossing to coat. Cover and cook for 5-6 minutes, stirring once or twice, until soft.

4. Add uncooked quinoa to vegetables and stir for 1-2 minutes, allowing it to lightly toast.

5. Pour in stock or water and bring the mixture to a boil. Immediately reduce to a simmer, cover and cook for 15 minutes until quinoa is cooked through. While quinoa is cooking, prepare eggs as you'd desire.

6. Once cooked, taste and season to your liking.

7. Serve quinoa in bowls topped with eggs and cooked bacon.

Almond Pancakes

These are a delicious alternative to regular pancakes. The almond flour is an excellent healthy fat. Better for blood sugar control. They are also low in carbs.

1 cup almond flour
1/4 cup water
2 eggs
1 tablespoon maple syrup

1/4 teaspoon salt
1 teaspoon oil as needed
(Optional) 1/2 teaspoon cinnamon, cardamom, nutmeg

1. Whisk almond flour, water, eggs, maple syrup, and salt together in a bowl until batter is smooth.

2. Heat oil in a skillet over medium heat; drop batter by large spoonfuls onto the griddle and cook until bubbles form and the edges are dry, 3 to 5 minutes. Be careful of the heat. These pancakes are high in healthy fat and easy to burn.

3. Flip, and cook until browned on the other side, 3 to 5 minutes.

4. Repeat with remaining batter.

Serve with cut up fresh fruit.

Chia Seed Breakfast Pudding

1 cup almond (or coconut) milk
1/4 cup chia seeds
Pure vanilla extract

Honey or stevia to taste
1/4 cup fruit (like raspberries, strawberries or kiwi)

Servings: 1

1. In a small Mason jar, stir together 1 cup almond milk and 1/4 cup chia seeds.

2. Add a splash of pure vanilla extract and a drizzle of honey and stir well until combined.

3. Transfer to the refrigerator and let sit until chia expands, about 8 hours.

4. When ready to eat, stir well, making sure to incorporate any clumps of chia. Feel free to get creative with your toppings or work with the fruit, spices, nuts or jams you have on hand.

    Some good ideas include:
        Chopped pear and walnuts
        Chopped apples with cinnamon and nutmeg
        Chopped almonds, ½ banana and unsweetened cocoa

Gluten-Free Pumpkin Muffins

These muffins are hearty, low sugar and delicious. You can bake them on the weekend and store them in the freezer for a quick breakfast on the go. Try substituting mashed squash such as delicata or butternut.

1 cup blanched almond flour
1 cup gluten-free oatmeal
1 teaspoon baking soda
1/2 teaspoon sea salt
2 teaspoons pumpkin pie spice
1 teaspoon cinnamon
1/4 teaspoon each: nutmeg, allspice,
    cloves

1 cup pumpkin puree
3 eggs
1/4 cup organic avocado oil, coconut or
    olive oil
1/4 cup maple syrup
1 cup chopped nuts (1/2 for topping)
1/2 cup raisins
1/2 cup coconut, unsweetened

Servings: about 18 muffins

1. Preheat oven to 350° F. Prepare muffin tins with muffin liners.
2. Mix dry ingredients together in a medium bowl, being sure to remove lumps.
3. Mix wet ingredients together in a large bowl.
4. Add dry ingredients to the wet ingredients and combine.
5. Pour batter into muffin tin, about 3/4 cup full for each.
6. Bake for 30 minutes or until a knife inserted in the middle comes out clean.

Avocado Toast

A quick, easy to make delight.

1 slice of GF hearty bread (I like 3 Bakers Ancient Grain or Udi's Chia and Millet)
1/2 ripe avocado plus a Good pinch of salt

1. Toast bread.
2. Meanwhile cut the avocado in half. Remove pit and use a large spoon to remove half of the avocado from the skin.
3. Mash the avocado with a fork until desired consistency.
4. Add salt
5. Spread avocado on toast. You can eat as is or add some toppings such as fresh herbs, tomatoes, garlic powder or an egg — fried, poached or soft cooked.

Breakfast Egg Cups (TO GO)

6 large eggs
2 tablespoons water
1 to 2 teaspoons olive oil
1/2 cup fresh spinach leaves

1/3 cup mushrooms, sliced
2 green onions, sliced
Salt and pepper to taste

Servings: 6

1. Preheat the oven to 350°F. Grease a muffin pan with cooking spray.

2. In a large bowl, whisk together the eggs, water and a pinch each of salt and pepper.

3. Stir in the spinach, mushrooms and green onions.

4. Divide the mixture evenly between 6 muffin pan cups. Bake for about 20 minutes, or until the muffins are set and firm in the center.

5. Remove the muffins from the oven and allow them to cool for 5 minutes in the pan, then use a butter knife to loosen the muffins from the cups.

6. Serve warm or room temperature.

Note: You can freeze the egg cups and pop them out of the freezer and go. A couple hours later they will be room temperature.

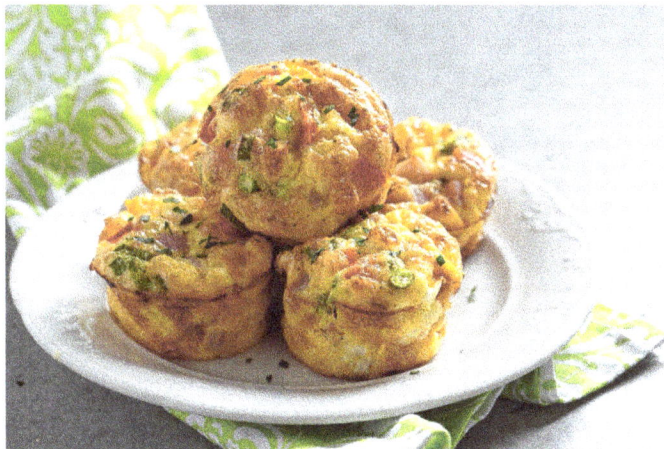

Healthy Homemade Granola

4 cups raw, gluten-free whole rolled oats
   (aka old fashion oats)
1 cup raw nuts, chopped
1/2 to 1 cup raw seeds, mixed (sunflower
   or pumpkin seeds are great)
2 tablespoons chia seeds and or flax
   seeds

1/2 cup unsweetened dried fruit, chopped
   (optional)
2 tablespoons grade-b maple syrup
2 tablespoons virgin coconut oil, melted
2 teaspoons cinnamon
1/2 teaspoon vanilla extract
1 large pinch fine sea salt

Servings: 4-6

1. Preheat the oven to 300° F.

2. Combine all ingredients on a baking sheet and use your clean hands to mix well and toss to coat. If you prefer a spatula works well, too.

3. Spread the mixture in a thin layer on a baking sheet and bake for 10-20 minutes, until very lightly toasted. Cool before serving or storing.

This granola can be kept in an airtight container in a cool, dry place for up to 2 weeks.

Note: Be creative with the ingredients. I use a mix of nuts, but you might like pecans with dried cherries, walnuts with cranberries, apricots with almonds, or dates with hazelnuts.

Hot Quinoa Breakfast Cereal with Fruit

1/2 cup quinoa, uncooked
1½ cups water
2 medium apples or pears (or really any fruit—peaches and nectarines are good, too)

1 to 2 teaspoons cinnamon, according to taste
1/4 cup chopped almonds, pecans or walnuts
Honey (optional)

1. Core or remove the stone of fruit. Chop into bite-sized pieces.

2. Add quinoa, water and fruit to a saucepan. Bring to a boil, cover and reduce to simmer for 20 - 25 minutes. The fruit will be soft, and the quinoa will have absorbed the water.

3. Stir in cinnamon and transfer mixture to two bowls.

4. Top with nuts.

5. Drizzle with a tiny bit of honey (optional), sprinkle with additional cinnamon and/or unsweetened shredded coconut (if desired).

Veggie Omelet

2 teaspoons olive oil
1/4 onion, peeled and chopped
1/4 red pepper, chopped
1/4 cup sliced mushrooms

1 cup loosely packed spinach leaves
2 eggs
1 tablespoon water
Salt and pepper

Servings: 1

1. In 4-inch nonstick skillet, heat oil over medium-high heat. Add bell pepper, onion and mushrooms to oil. Cook 2 minutes, stirring frequently, until onion is tender. Stir in spinach; continue cooking and stirring just until spinach wilts.

2. In medium bowl, beat eggs, water, salt and pepper with fork or whisk until well mixed. Pour egg mixture into pan. Let the eggs set a little bit. Using a spatula, lift the sides of the omelet and tilt the pan so the liquid on top flows to the bottom of the pan. Continue this process until the top of the omelet is cooked.

3. Fold the omelet and flip to the opposite side for a bit to lightly brown bottom of omelet. Do not overcook as the omelet will continue cooking.

4. Gently slide out of pan onto plate. Serve immediately.

DESSERTS

I am not a huge fan of desserts largely because eating sugar only feeds cravings. But occasionally we all love a good dessert. The recipes here are made with reduced sugar.

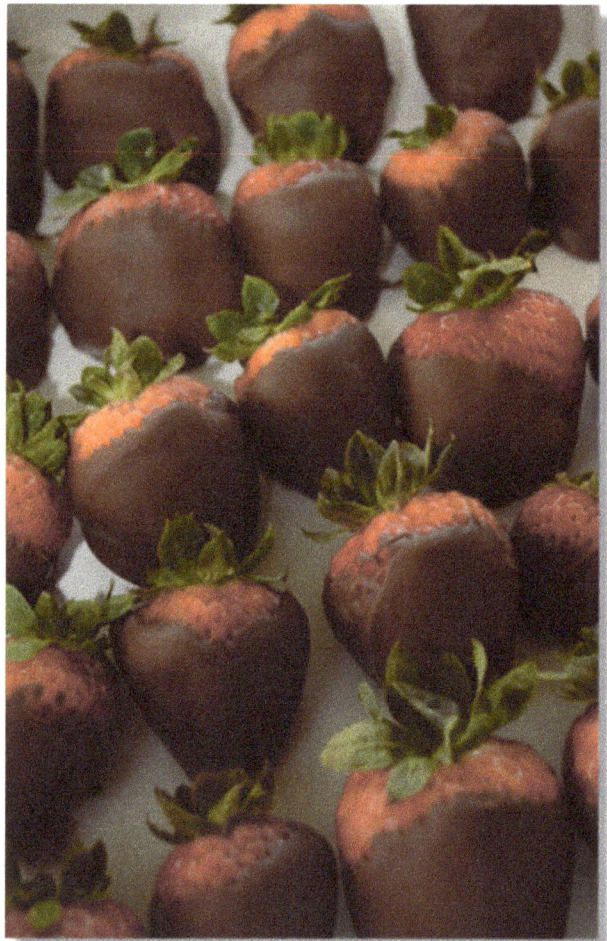

Coconut "Cookies"

2 tablespoons unsweetened almond milk
   (or other non-dairy milk)
3 tablespoons virgin coconut oil
2 tablespoons unsweetened cacao
   powder
1/2 cup unsweetened shredded coconut
1 cup rolled oats (gluten free for GF
   eaters)

1/3 cup salted natural almond butter,
   crunchy or creamy (or cashew butter)
1/2 teaspoon pure vanilla extract
pinch sea salt
Drops of stevia to taste
2 tablespoons crushed salted almonds
   peanuts or shredded coconut (for
   topping)

1. Line a baking sheet with parchment or wax paper.
2. Add almond milk, cocoa powder and coconut oil to a medium saucepan, over medium heat and bring to melt over medium low heat, stirring frequently.
3. Remove from heat. Add almond butter, oats, shredded coconut, vanilla and salt plus stevia to taste.
4. Stir to combine and fully incorporate all ingredients.
5. Drop heaping tablespoons of the batter onto the prepared baking sheet and sprinkle with crushed almonds and/or additional flaked coconut (optional).
6. Let sit at room temperature until cooled and hardened - about 25-30 minutes.
7. Keep in the refrigerator for up to 3 days, though best when fresh.

Chocolate Dipped Banana Bites

2 tablespoons dark chocolate chips
1 small banana, peeled and cut into 1-inch chunks

1. Place chocolate in a small microwave safe bowl and microwave for 30 seconds.
2. Dip banana in chocolate. Let it set and serve.

Note: You can make this with strawberries, pineapple, pears—just use your imagination.

Dark Chocolate Coconut Bites

2 cups coconut, unsweetened
4 tablespoons honey or maple syrup
5 tablespoons virgin coconut oil

1 teaspoon vanilla
4 ounces dark chocolate for melting (i.e. chocolate chips)

1. In a blender or food processor pulse the coconut until the texture becomes like flour. Transfer to a bowl and add the honey or maple syrup, coconut oil, and vanilla. Stir until a thick batter forms.

2. Using your hands, squeeze the mixture into about 18 small balls. You may need to knead the batter a bit to get them to roll them into balls. Place the coconut balls in the refrigerator for about 30 minutes or until firm.

3. Melt the chocolate slowly and gently until smooth and spreadable. You can either do this in a microwave or by melting the chocolate in a double boiler.

4. Lay out a sheet of wax paper. Using two forks, roll each coconut ball in the chocolate until completely covered. Let the extra chocolate drip off the fork. Place the chocolate covered ball onto wax paper and chill until the chocolate has hardened. Store in the refrigerator.

Chocolate Avocado Pudding

Creamy, cool and delish. A good way to get a serving of healthy fat.

2 avocados (large & ripe)
1/2 cup raw cacao powder
2 teaspoons vanilla extract

1/4 cup plant-based milk, unsweetened
1/4 cup maple syrup or a couple of drops of liquid stevia

1. Slice the avocados, discard the pit and skins and add to the bowl of a food processor.

2. Add the cacao powder, vanilla extract, sweetener and plant milk and process together until smooth. Transfer to a bowl, tightly cover and refrigerate until set, about 30 minutes or so.

Note: For variety, you can add essential oils (certified pure therapeutic grade, e.g., *doTerra*) for flavoring. Delete the vanilla add peppermint or wild orange.

Cranberry-Apple Crisp

Filling:
- 4 large apples
- 2 cups cranberries
- 2 tablespoons brown sugar
- 1 tablespoon all-purpose flour, gluten free
- 1 tablespoon fresh lemon juice

Topping:
- 1/3 cup all-purpose flour, gluten free
- 1/2 cup regular oats, gluten free
- 1/4 cup brown sugar
- 2 teaspoons ground cinnamon
- 4 tablespoons grass-fed butter, chilled and cut into small piece

1. Preheat oven to 375° F.
2. Combine the filling ingredients and spoon into a 13" x 9" baking dish.
3. Combine the flour, brown sugar, oats and cinnamon. Cut in the butter with a pastry blender or 2 knives until the consistency of coarse meal.
4. Bake in the oven for 30-40 minutes or until bubbly and the apples are soft.

Blueberry and Raspberry Crisp

Filling:
- 4 cups blueberries
- 2 cups raspberries
- 2 tablespoons maple syrup
- 1 tablespoon all-purpose flour, gluten free
- 1 tablespoon fresh lemon juice

Topping:
- 1/3 cup all-purpose flour, gluten free
- 1/2 cup regular oats, gluten free
- 1/4 cup brown sugar
- 2 teaspoons ground cinnamon
- 4 tablespoons grass-fed butter, chilled and cut into small pieces – or use coconut oil to keep it dairy-free

1. Preheat oven to 375° F.
2. Combine the filling ingredients and spoon into a 13" x 9" baking dish.
3. Combine the flour, brown sugar, oats and cinnamon. Cut in the butter with a pastry blender or 2 knives until the consistency of coarse meal.
4. Bake in the oven for 30 minutes or until bubbly.

Healthy Ginger-Pumpkin Mousse

1 avocado
1 sliced and frozen banana, thawed for 5
* minutes*
3/4 cup canned pure pumpkin puree

2 tablespoons pure maple syrup
1/2 teaspoon ground pumpkin pie spice
1/4 teaspoon ginger

Optional Topping: Super Seed Topping
Servings: 4

1. Place the avocado, banana, pumpkin, maple syrup, and pumpkin pie spice in the bowl of a food processor and process 30 seconds.

2. Stop and scrape down the sides of the bowl. Continue to process until smooth and creamy, about 1 more minute. The mixture should resemble mousse or pudding.

3. Meanwhile, for the topping, see Super Seed Topping in Sauces & Dressings.

4. Scoop the mousse into 4 bowls and sprinkle evenly with the topping.

Wild Orange Dark Chocolate-Dipped Strawberries

A cinch to make and an elegant healthy dessert.

2 3.5 oz. bars of Lindt 85% Dark Chocolate
1 pound of strawberries with stems, washed and dried well
1 drop of doTERRA Wild Orange Essential oil*
Servings: 4-6

1. Put the dark chocolate in a heatproof medium bowl. Fill a medium saucepan with a couple inches of water and bring to a simmer over medium heat. Turn off the heat; set the bowl of chocolate over the water to melt. Stir until smooth.

    You can also melt the chocolate in a microwave at half power, for 1 minute, stir and then heat for another minute or until melted.

2. Add a drop of *doTerra* Wild Orange to the chocolate

3. Once the chocolate is melted and smooth, remove from the heat. Line a sheet pan with parchment or waxed paper. Holding the strawberry by the stem, dip the fruit into the dark chocolate, lift and twist slightly, letting any excess chocolate fall back into the bowl. Place strawberries on parchment paper. Repeat with the rest of the strawberries.

4. Set the strawberries aside until the chocolate sets, about 30 minutes.

*Make sure to always use a certified pure therapeutic grade oil (CPTG) such as *doTERRA* for ingestion.

Chocolate Cherry Bars

1/2 cups raw walnuts
3/4 cup raw almonds
1/4 cup Medjool dates, pitted
1/2 cup dried blueberries
1 teaspoon vanilla extract

1/8 teaspoon ground cinnamon
1 cup dried cherries
2 tablespoons cacao nibs
1 tablespoon coconut oil, unrefined

1. In a food processor, combine the walnuts and the almonds, and process the nuts into the size of small gravel.

2. Add the dates, berries, vanilla extract and cinnamon powder, and process until the mixture forms clumps and begins to stick together.

3. Add the cherries, cacao nibs and coconut oil. Process briefly to incorporate the ingredients but leave some small chunks for texture.

4. Stop the machine and check the consistency. Depending on the natural moisture of the dates, you may need to add a touch of water or coconut oil 1 teaspoon at a time to get the crumbs to stick together when pinched.

5. If the dough is too wet, blend in a few extra almonds.

6. Place the dough on a large sheet of plastic wrap on a cutting board. Press the dough into a compact rectangle, then wrap it tightly in the plastic, compacting it even more.

7. Use a rolling pin to roll the dough into a 1-inch-thick layer.

8. Unwrap the dough and cut it into bars or bites as desired.

Note: Energy bars will last several weeks unrefrigerated and covered or keep them in the freezer for long-term storage.

SELECT DAIRY RECIPES

This section is for those of you who don't need to avoid dairy. These are some of my all-time favorites!

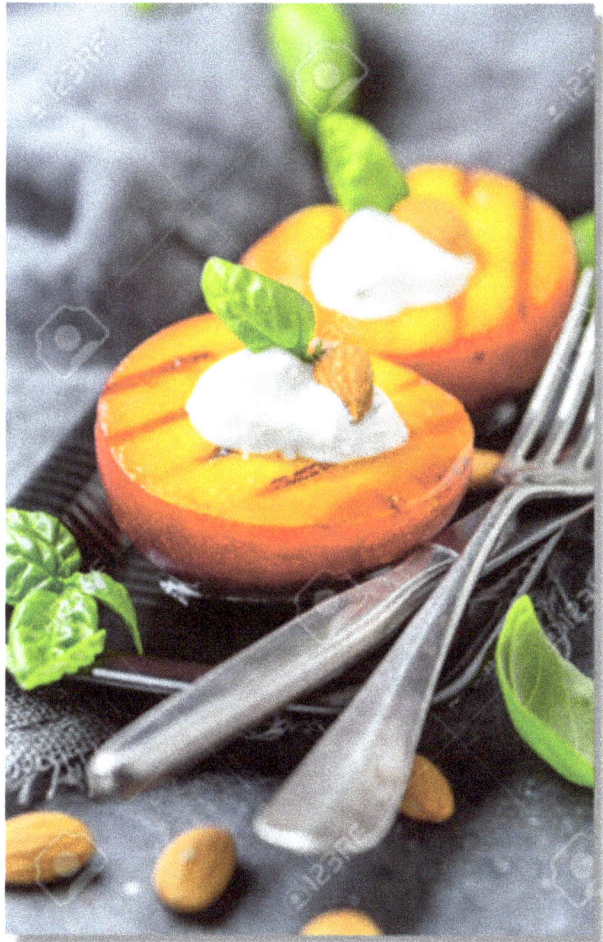

Farro Salad with Peas, Asparagus and Feta

Farro is a delicious nutty-tasting ancient grain. This is a great salad for the spring, but you can make it autumn and winter hardy by using kale, Brussels sprouts and winter squash instead of the spring vegetables and using rosemary or thyme as an herb.

1½ cups farro
12 ounces asparagus, trimmed, cut into 1
  1/2-inch lengths
1 8-ounce package peas, snow, or sugar
  snap peas
12 ounces grape tomatoes, halved

1/2 cup thinly sliced and chopped red
  onion
6 tablespoons chopped fresh dill
1/2 cup olive oil
1/4 cup Sherry wine vinegar
1 7-ounce package feta cheese, crumbled

1. Cook farro in large saucepan of boiling salted water until just tender, about 25 to 30 minutes. Drain. Transfer to large bowl.

2. Meanwhile, steam asparagus and sugar snap peas in another saucepan until crisp-tender, about 3 to 5 minutes. Drain. Add to farro with tomatoes, onion, and dill.

3. Whisk oil and vinegar in small bowl. Season dressing with salt and pepper. Add dressing and feta to salad; toss to coat and serve.

Polenta Bake with Shrimp

1 16 oz. tube of gluten free polenta
1 lb. peeled and deveined large raw
  shrimp
1 cup cherry tomatoes, halved
2 tablespoons olive oil

1/2 teaspoon salt
1/2 teaspoon pepper, or to taste
3 oz. parmesan cheese, grated
1/2 teaspoon paprika
2 tablespoons sliced scallions

1. Preheat oven to 400° F. Slice the polenta into even slices about ¼" thick. Place in an oven proof casserole.
2. Mix the shrimp, tomatoes, olive oil, salt, pepper and paprika. Layer on top of the polenta. Bake until the shrimp are just cooked through, about 5 to 7 minutes. The time will depend on how large the shrimp are.
3. Sprinkle with scallions and parmesan cheese and serve.

Asparagus Quinoa Salad

Serve warm as a side dish, or chilled as an Asparagus salad.

1-2 bunches asparagus
1 cup quinoa (uncooked)
1/2 cup red onion, chopped
1/2 cup kalamata olives (pitted, sliced)

1/2 cup feta
1/2 cup toasted pine nuts (optional)
Handful Italian parsley or cilantro
Zest from one lemon

Dressing:

1/3 cup olive oil
3 tablespoons whole grain mustard
2 tablespoons red wine vinegar

2 tablespoons lemon juice
1 teaspoon salt
1 teaspoon pepper

Servings: 4-6

1. Heat oven to 425° F.

2. Trim off the tough ends of the asparagus. Lay them on a baking sheet and drizzle with 1-2 tablespoons olive oil, sprinkle with a generous pinch of salt and cracked pepper, and half of the lemon zest. Roast in the oven until just tender, about 20-25 minutes. Cut into bite size pieces.

3. Bring 2 cups of salted water to a boil. Add 1 cup quinoa and cook until al dente about 20 minutes.

4. While quinoa is cooking, make the dressing. In a small bowl, stir all dressing ingredients together.

5. Place quinoa in a large bowl. Toss it with the dressing, olives, red onion, asparagus, feta, pine nuts, fresh herbs and lemon zest. Serve warm, or chill and serve as a salad.

Eggplant Bundles

These are especially great at the peak of the summer harvest when eggplant, peppers, tomatoes, fresh herbs and summer squash are at their best. You can serve the bundles with a gluten free grain like quinoa and dinner is done. Because you are using the grill, cleanup is a cinch too.

1 large eggplant
Salt and freshly ground pepper to taste
1/4 cup dry red wine
1/4 cup fig balsamic vinegar—
   unflavored is fine
1 tablespoon honey
1 small yellow squash
1 small zucchini

1 large red pepper, seeded and quartered
2 tablespoons extra virgin olive oil
1/2 cup (4 ounces) goat cheese
2 tablespoons fresh basil, chopped—plus
   some for garnish
1 teaspoon fresh oregano, chopped
1 cup cherry tomatoes, cut in half

1. Combine the red wine, balsamic vinegar and honey in a saucepan over medium high heat. Bring to a boil and reduce heat to medium. Simmer until reduced in half (¼ cup). Set aside.

2. Prepare grill to a medium heat.

3. Prepare vegetables: Trim ends from squash and slice lengthwise into ¼ in slices. Cut the eggplant crosswise into at least eight ½" slices. Flatten the pepper quarters by hand. Brush the vegetable with the olive oil and season with salt and pepper.

4. Combine cheese, basil and oregano and season with salt and pepper.

5. Grill eggplant and pepper 3 to 5 minutes per side and the squash 2 to 3 per side. Each piece should have grill marks and be soft and pliable.

6. Assemble the bundles: Place eggplant slice on a plate and top with ¼ of the cheese mixture. Lay one strip of summer squash and one of zucchini side by side. Drizzle with about a teaspoon of wine sauce. Next layer is the pepper. Top it all off with an eggplant slice and drizzle again with 2 teaspoons of sauce. Repeat for the remaining 3 bundles.

7. Garnish with cherry tomatoes and basil.

Grilled Peaches with Mascarpone Cheese

Olive oil
3 firm but ripe peaches, pitted, halved
2 tablespoons sugar or stevia to taste
2 tablespoons brandy

1 tablespoon fresh lemon juice
1/2 cup mascarpone cheese, room
* temperature*
1/4 teaspoon vanilla extract

Servings: 6

1. Place a grill pan over medium-high heat or prepare the barbecue (medium-high heat). Lightly brush the grill pan or rack with oil. Place the peaches on the grill pan and do not move the peaches, otherwise you will not have those great grill marks. It takes about 2 to 3 minutes per side to get those grill marks.

2. Grill the peaches until the grill marks are formed, slightly softened and heated through, about 5 to 6 minutes total.

3. Meanwhile, stir the sugar, brandy, and lemon juice in a medium bowl to blend. Set the brandy mixture aside.

4. As the peaches are ready, remove them from the grill and place them in a shallow baking dish. Top them with the brandy mixture and toss gently to coat. Set aside for 15 minutes and allow to marinate, tossing occasionally.

5. Meanwhile, stir the mascarpone and vanilla in a small bowl to blend.

6. Divide the grilled peach mixture equally among 6 coupe dishes. Dollop the mascarpone mixture atop the peaches and serve.

Chickpea Crust Pizza

I love this pizza crust because it is high in fiber and chock full of slow carbs. Whatever veggie and/or herbs that are fresh and in season would be good choices for toppings. Other toppings include sundried tomatoes and kalamata olives.

1 cup chickpea flour, freshly ground if
    you can—I use a spice grinder
1 cup warm water
1/4 cup olive oil, divided
2 garlic cloves, pressed or minced
1/2 teaspoon sea salt
1/4 teaspoon pepper

1/2 tablespoon of fresh rosemary,
    minced
1/2 cup pizza sauce
1/2 cup shredded mozzarella
Handful of baby spinach
Sliced mushrooms
Very finely sliced onion

1. In a bowl, whisk together the chickpea flour, warm water, 2 tablespoons of the olive oil, garlic and salt. Let the mixture rest at room temperature for at least 30 minutes. The batter should have the consistency of thick cream.

2. Preheat the oven to 450° F. Place a 10-inch cast iron skillet in the oven to preheat when you are ready to make the pizza {12-inch skillet is OK).

3. Add 1 tablespoon olive oil to the pan and swirl the pan around so the oil is evenly distributed. Pour in the chickpea batter and return the skillet to the oven. Cook for 12 to 15 minutes, until the crust is set, and the edges are pulling away from the sides of the pan. If the top is not brown, increase the heat to broil and place the crust a few inches below the broiler to brown it up a bit.

4. Turn off broiler and turn oven to 425° F.

5. Spread the remaining 1 tablespoon olive oil on top of the crust (it will soak right in). Top the crust with pizza sauce and mozzarella, and other toppings.

6. Return the skillet to the oven and bake for 8 to 10 minutes, until the cheese is browning and the socca is crisp.

7. Remove from oven and sprinkle fresh thyme on top. Let the pizza cool for 2 to 3 minutes before slicing into 4 pieces and serving.

Light Chicken Verde Nachos

5 corn tortillas
1 tablespoon extra-virgin olive oil plus
   olive oil to spray
1/2 lb. chicken breasts, thinly sliced
   lengthwise and crosswise into strips
1 small red onion diced

1 16 oz. jar salsa verde
1 cup cherry tomatoes, halved
2 oz. queso fresco crumbled
1 avocado chopped
1/2 cup cilantro roughly chopped

Servings: 2

1. Preheat your oven to 400° F. Stack the tortillas and cut them all into 6 wedges each for a total of 30 wedges. Arrange the pieces on a baking sheet and spray them generously with olive oil. Bake for 15-18 minutes until the chips are all crisp. Cool chips to room temperature.

2. Add the oil to a medium saucepan over medium heat. Cook the chicken and onion for 3-5 minutes. Add the salsa verde. Cook the mixture for 5 to 8 minutes, until the salsa verde reduces to about half the volume and the chicken is no longer pink in the center.

3. On a large plate arrange the baked chips and top with the chicken verde mixture, tomatoes, queso fresco, avocado and cilantro. Serve immediately.

Smoked Trout Mousse

1 cup mascarpone cheese
1 cup coarsely flaked smoked trout
2 tablespoons prepared horseradish,
   drained

2 tablespoons chopped scallions
1 tablespoon chopped fresh dill
2 teaspoons lemon juice

1. Place the mascarpone cheese in a bowl. Fold in half the trout, then the horseradish, scallions, dill, and lemon juice.

2. Season with salt and pepper. Fold in the remaining trout. Chill.

3. Serve on cucumber slices. Pumpernickel bread toast points are good too if gluten is not an issue.

Spring Vegetable Egg Casserole with Cheese

This easy casserole is great for brunch, but I love it for dinner, too.

1 tablespoon olive oil
1/2 cup diced yellow onion
2 cups asparagus, cut into 1-inch pieces
6 cups packed fresh spinach leaves
2 cloves garlic, minced
2 tablespoons freshly chopped dill
4 green onions, sliced

½ cup cheese: gouda, edam, Havarti
 are all great choices
12 large eggs, whisked
1/2 cup reduced fat milk
Salt and black pepper, to taste
½ cup feta cheese

Servings: 10-12

1. Preheat oven to 350° F. Spray or brush a 9×13 inch baking dish with olive oil.

2. In a large skillet, heat olive oil over high heat. Add the onion and cook until tender, about 3 minutes. Stir in the asparagus, spinach, and garlic. Cook for 4 minutes, or until vegetables are tender and spinach is wilted. Stir in the dill, the gouda cheese and the green onions.

3. Season with salt and black pepper, to taste. Pour vegetable mixture into prepared baking dish and spread out evenly.

4. In a medium bowl, combine eggs and milk. Whisk well. Season with salt and black pepper, to taste. Pour egg mixture evenly over the veggies. Sprinkle feta cheese on top.

5. Bake for 30-35 minutes or until eggs are set and slightly golden around the edges. A knife inserted into the center should come out clean. Remove from oven and let cool for 10 minutes. Cut into squares and serve warm.

Note: This casserole reheats well and can be made a day in advance. Or make it the night before right through step 4 and pop it in the oven the next day.

Acknowledgements

The primary motivation and inspiration to write this book came from my clients. It started by helping them to have an easy way to integrate the concepts about food and nutrition that we discussed in our coaching sessions. Sharing recipes that I had collected and curated over the last 30 years. Then I started to get great feedback about the recipes particularly about the uniqueness of the ingredients and the use of herbs, spices and other flavorings. This created the spark. I am in deep gratitude to all my clients who have provided feedback and support.

My friend, Robin Eichert was insightful when she recommended on one of our Friday morning hikes that the book include meal plans to help my readers even more. I liked this idea with a little bit of reticence because I am not a fan of telling people what to eat. To me, it can be too much like a diet. It works better to inspire good choices. Over time these evolved into menus based on mindfulness from feedback from other friends, particularly Missi Blake who came up with the name Mindful Menus.

Others who helped with the book, include my close friends Kate Stordy and Mary Burnett. They both took time out of their busy lives to read the entire book and gave me smart constructive feedback.

My good friend and neighbor, Selinda Chiquoine did an expert job of proofing and editing even though she got the transcript at the very last moment and never complained at all.

Marisa Imon, a new friend, was an inspiration, too. She has already published a book so could give me some good tips and pointers not to mention moral support. She gave selflessly of her time.

Finally, this book would have never become a reality without my husband, Karl Wendelowski. He provided amazing technical support, smart project management and a ton of thoughtful feedback. I can tell you, there were plenty of nights when he didn't get much sleep!

Writing a book can be very similar to helping a person heal. It takes a village.

About Ruth

Ruth Clark, RD, MPH is a board certified Registered Dietitian and functional nutritionist with a master's degree in Public Health and more than 35 years of experience in the nutrition field. She specializes in helping mid-life and older women who are struggling with weight, fatigue, chronic pain, and mood issues to create more vitality in their lives.

Ruth has held positions at both Harvard and Tufts teaching hospitals, in corporate America, and was formerly Executive Director of Wellness Programming for the Deaconess Hospital in Boston. She is a nationally known nutrition lecturer, and a former member of the Scientific Advisory Board for several nutrition companies. Ruth is also the creator of the successful Rejuvenation Jump Start program.

www.smartnutritionllc.com
ruth@ruthrd,com

www.ingramcontent.com/pod-product-compliance
Lightning Source LLC
Chambersburg PA
CBHW080359030426
42334CB00024B/2925